It's Easy *to Be* Healthy

It's Easy *to Be* Healthy

Malaika's Guide to Living a Good Life

Malaika Arora

BLOOMSBURY
NEW DELHI • LONDON • OXFORD • NEW YORK • SYDNEY

BLOOMSBURY INDIA
Bloomsbury Publishing India Pvt. Ltd
Second Floor, LSC Building No. 4, DDA Complex, Pocket C – 6 & 7,
Vasant Kunj, New Delhi, 110070

BLOOMSBURY, BLOOMSBURY INDIA and the Diana logo
are trademarks of Bloomsbury Publishing Plc

First published in India 2025

Copyright © Malaika Arora, 2025

Malaika Arora has asserted her moral rights to be identified as the author
of this work in accordance with the Indian Copyright Act, 1957

All rights reserved. No part of this publication may be: i) reproduced
or transmitted in any form, electronic or mechanical, including
photocopying, recording or by means of any information storage or
retrieval system without prior permission in writing from the publishers;
or ii) used or reproduced in any way for the training, development or
operation of artificial intelligence (AI) technologies, including generative
AI technologies. The rights holders expressly reserve this publication
from the text and data mining exception as per Article 4(3) of the Digital
Single Market Directive (EU) 2019/790

This book is not a substitute for medical attention, treatment, examination,
advice, treatment of existing conditions or diagnosis. It is not intended
to provide a clinical diagnosis nor take the place of medical advice from
a fully qualified medical practitioner. Consult your healthcare service
provider before following any health advice given in this book

ISBN: PB: 978-93-56405-43-1; eBook: 978-93-56405-42-4
2 4 6 8 10 9 7 5 3 1

Typeset in Fouriner by Manipal Technologies Limited
Printed and bound in India by Thomson Press India Ltd

To find out more about our authors and books visit www.bloomsbury.com
and sign up for our newsletters

Contents

How to Use This Book — vii

Introduction — 1

PART I: BEAUTY

1. Skin: Glow from the Inside Out — 15
2. Hair: The Crown You Never Take Off — 51
3. Magic Potion: Sleep, Water, Sunshine — 83

PART II: BODY

4. Food: Fuel for the Body and Mind — 109
5. Fitness: More Than Just a Look — 147
6. Women's Health: Navigating the Phases of Life — 190

PART III: MIND

7. Holistic Wellness: The Mind, Body, and Soul Connection — 213
8. Unapologetically Me: My Life, Unfiltered — 236

Conclusion — 262

About the Author — 269

How to Use This Book

This book isn't a rule book. It's not about chasing perfection or sticking to some rigid routine. It's more like a wellness companion – something you can turn to when you want a little clarity, inspiration, or even just a nudge to reset. Maybe you're curious about how I manage my skin and hair. Maybe you want to switch up your food habits. Or maybe, you're just looking for small ways to take better care of your mind. Wherever you are in your journey, you'll find little things here – rituals, meals, habits, reminders – that have helped me feel stronger, calmer, and more connected to myself.

You don't need to start at Chapter 1 or follow any particular sequence. This book is meant to be picked up, put down, bookmarked, scribbled in, and returned to whenever you feel the need. If you're looking for something specific – say, a fitness tip, a mood-lifting practice, or a quick health shot – you'll find it. Let the chapters meet you where you are.

The book is divided into three parts: **Beauty**, **Body**, and **Mind**. Each section focuses on a different aspect of well-being, but nothing in this space works in isolation. You'll notice some overlap – like how sleep shows up in skincare, stress relief, and strength-building. That's not by accident. Wellness doesn't exist in silos. One small shift can ripple through everything else.

Some of what I've shared is deeply personal. Some of it is light and simple. All of it is real. These are the routines I return to, the lessons I've learned through trial and error, and the practices that still ground me today. You'll see a few things repeated across chapters – not because we forgot to edit them out but because that's how they function in real life. When something works, it works across categories.

And just to be clear – I'm not a doctor or an expert. I'm sharing what I've lived, what I've tested, and what I believe in. If something speaks to you, try it. If it doesn't, skip it. Take what you need. Leave what you don't. Come back when you're ready. Most important, be kind to yourself along the way.

Because at the end of the day, that's what this is all about: feeling good, in ways that last.

Introduction

Hi, I'm Malaika Arora. Some of you might know me as the girl who danced on a moving train in the song 'Chaiyya Chaiyya' or lit up screens with 'Munni Badnaam Hui'. Maybe you've seen me judge talent shows like *India's Got Talent* and *Jhalak Dikhhla Jaa* or tuned in to my show *Moving in with Malaika*. But behind all the glitz and glamour, I'm someone who has been on a parallel journey – mastering not just my craft but also my body and mind.

The book you're holding in your hands is my way of sharing everything I've learned in my 25+ years in the entertainment business. I've always wanted to create something that feels personal, accessible, and empowering – whether you're looking for beauty tips, wellness rituals, or just a little inspiration to take better care of yourself. But before we dive into all the tips and tricks, let me take you back to where it all began.

From MTV to Munni

My journey was hardly a deliberate plan; it was more a series of serendipitous (and occasionally less fortunate) moments that unfolded unexpectedly. I've always believed that when opportunities come your way, you grab them with both hands and give it your all. That relentless drive to do it all, to push boundaries and challenge myself, has shaped everything I am today. When I started modelling in the early 1990s, my first gig was with *MTV Loveline*, which opened doors to a career I could not have dreamed of. From walking for legends like Rohit Bal, Wendell Rodricks, and Tarun Tahiliani to dancing my heart out on-screen – a love I'd nurtured since my ballet classes as a child – life felt like a whirlwind of possibilities. But as I stepped deeper into this world, I realized that it takes more than just talent to thrive – it takes resilience, discipline, and an unwavering commitment to self-care.

Take 'Chaiyya Chaiyya' for example. Balancing on top of a moving train in the heat, holding poses for endless retakes – it wasn't glamorous, but it taught me that the effort behind the scenes is what creates magic on-screen.

By the time I shot 'Kaal Dhamaal' in 2005, fresh out of postpartum recovery, the stakes felt even higher. I was grappling with hair fall, stretch marks, and a body that didn't feel like mine. Dancing again was both terrifying and liberating – a chance to prove to myself that I could embrace this new phase of life.

Introduction

And then came 'Munni Badnaam Hui', where I was in the better half of my thirties, more confident in my skin and my craft than ever. It was a reminder that age isn't a barrier to shining in a fiercely competitive industry.

People have often been kind with their words. I remember Shah Rukh once telling me, 'You don't just dance, you own the frame' – a compliment I've never forgotten. Salman, who's seen me on countless sets, used to call me one of the hardest-working people in the room. And Farah – who's choreographed so many of my most memorable songs – often says I'm living proof that you can rewrite your story, no matter the odds. These aren't just flattering lines. They're reminders of how far I've come, and how much work it's taken behind the scenes to get here.

Through these collaborations, I built a three-decade-long career alongside forging lifelong friendships. On days when the music wouldn't sync or when exhaustion set in, it was my work family that reminded me of my strength. Those were the moments that taught me what it means to truly 'show up' – for your team and for yourself.

Reinvention Is My Middle Name!

Each of these experiences taught me something new – not just about dancing or acting but about myself.

It wasn't just about the songs or the performances; it was about reinvention. Reinventing myself has been a constant thread in my life – from modelling to dancing, acting to entrepreneurship.

As fulfilling as my artistic journey has been, my role as an entrepreneur has been equally rewarding. Whether it's the Diva Yoga – a wellness studio empowering women to embrace health and mindfulness – or the Scarlett House – my first restaurant – every venture reflects my passion for promoting wellness as a lifestyle. From recipes inspired by my own kitchen to yoga programmes that helped me heal, these ventures are extensions of my belief that small, intentional steps can lead to incredible shifts.

Although my entrepreneurial side is not known to many, fitness has always been a cornerstone of my life – a journey shaped by diverse experiences: hours spent perfecting dance routines, intense gym sessions, and exploring holistic therapies. Yoga became a turning point in my twenties after a dance injury kept me from the gym. What began as a necessity turned into a passion, eventually forming the core of my wellness routine. But my approach to fitness has never been limited to one practice. Dancing taught me rhythm and discipline, gym sessions pushed my physical boundaries, and holistic therapies showed me the power of nurturing the mind and body together. Yoga, in particular, taught me to listen to my body – to honour its limitations and celebrate its strength. It's about more than physical recovery; it's about creating harmony in life's chaos and finding balance, both within and beyond the mat.

And yet, there have been moments that tested me.

In 2022, a car accident shook me to my core. Recovery wasn't just physical; it was emotional too. I had to confront my fears, slow down, and, in many ways, start anew. That experience reaffirmed what yoga had already taught me years ago: the body is incredibly resilient, and with the right care, it can heal, adapt, and thrive. In retrospect, that accident changed something deep within me. It made me face my fears head-on, and now I feel I have no fears left. It's given me a kind of fearlessness I didn't know I was capable of – a drive to take on everything I'd been hesitant about before. Whether it's doing stand-up on-stage or adding more feathers to my hat, I've realized that life's too short to hold back.

From the Big Four-Oh to the Big Five-Oh!

Looking back, my forties have been a transformational phase for me. Honestly, it wasn't until I hit 40 that I felt like I was truly coming into my own. There's something about that age – a point when society starts whispering that women should slow down or fade away. I felt the opposite. I felt unstoppable, like I was just getting started.

It wasn't just about age; it was about everything I had been through by then. My fourth decade brought its fair share of setbacks – a divorce, heartbreaks, break-ups, and moments of profound doubt. But those challenges also shaped me. For years, I had lived trying to make others happy, putting myself second or even last. Only in my forties did I finally decide it was time to do things for myself – to live my dreams and confront my fears.

By then, I had spent years trying and testing everything under the sun – diets, therapies, workout regimes – and while some worked, others didn't. What mattered was that I kept going. I had been through too much to continue second-guessing myself. Really, how sad would I be if I sat and questioned if that troll who called me an 'aunty' was right? Instead, I began to trust my instincts more. And found joy in knowing that I am that 'aunty' who can out-thumka them on the dance floor any day! I finally started appreciating my body for everything it had carried me through – the triumphs, the setbacks, and even the scars.

Introduction

I see this time as a decade of reinvention. It wasn't easy, but it was worth it. Every experience, whether good or bad, became a stepping stone. From trying my hand at stand-up comedy to re-entering the dating world, it was a decade where I realized that the only limits we have are the ones we place on ourselves. For someone who has worked all her life, I've never felt more energetic, more willing to grab opportunities, and more excited about what lies ahead.

And now, as I turn 50, that fire hasn't dimmed one bit. If anything, it burns brighter. This new chapter isn't about fearing ageing – it's about embracing the wisdom and confidence that comes with it. Today, I can proudly say that I am my biggest cheerleader, and I refuse to let anyone or anything hold me back.

At some point, I realized that this journey of self-care wasn't just about looking good – it was about feeling good. It wasn't just about mastering dance moves or maintaining a schedule – it was about finding balance in the chaos. And that road hasn't been easy. It's been filled with twists and turns, from injuries that stymied me to trolls who tried to shame me. I've been called names, judged for prioritizing myself (while being super transparent about it), and even labelled a 'bad mother'.

From Me to You: Here's Why

Through all these experiences, one question has followed me: 'How do you do it all?' Whether it's staying fit, managing a packed schedule, or showing up with energy and poise, people are always curious about my so-called secrets. And I get it – it's easy to assume that actors are somehow born this way, that we're 'gifted' with glowing skin, perfect hair, and boundless energy. But let me tell you, that's far from the truth.

I wasn't born with flawless skin or a fiery metabolism. My weight has fluctuated, my skin has broken out, and my hair has thinned – just like anyone else's. I don't think what sets me apart is luck; I believe it's just consistency. Over the years, I've tried countless routines, diets, skincare products, and holistic therapies. Some things worked; others didn't. But through it all, what stayed with me was the discipline to show up for myself every single day.

After three decades of trial and error, what I've found is a way of living that works for me – and that's exactly why I decided to write this book. I wanted to put it all down in one place – from the elixirs and health shots I swear by to the little habits and rituals that make a big difference.

Introduction

So I finally decided to put pen to paper and share the truth (with whoever's interested!) – no filters, no pretences, just everything that has shaped my wellness journey. Writing this book feels like a cumulative effect of everything I've lived through – moments of doubt, discovery, and acceptance.

This isn't a manual on perfection. I'm not here to tell you to follow a strict regimen or to avoid that slice of cake. Instead, I want to show you how simple it can be to feel good. Being healthy doesn't mean undertaking gruelling gym sessions, being tied to the weighing scale, or following impossible diets. It means learning how to balance – listening to your body, knowing when to rest, and giving yourself grace. Ayurveda and yoga aren't just trends for me – they are lifelines that keep me grounded. Discipline (not to be confused with restriction) is at the core of how I live, and it's one of the biggest lessons I hope to share with you. You'll read about my daily rituals, the little things that keep me grounded – from morning affirmations to sunbathing, fasting to indulging, and movement to mindfulness.

I also want to break the silence and normalize discussions around women's health – the conversations we shy away from most. Let's talk about the real stuff – pregnancy, postpartum recovery, perimenopause, and menopause. These topics are still treated like taboos when they're as natural as breathing. Whether it's mental wellness, hormonal changes, or simply carving out time for regular check-ups, it's time we stop tiptoeing around these topics. As women, we're often told to put everyone else first. And while that instinct is beautiful, it's also exhausting. I've been guilty of it too. But here's what I've learned – you can't pour from an empty cup.

I want to demystify a lot of myths around beauty and health, and among the biggest ones is the idea that self-care is selfish. The truth? It's necessary! Taking care of your health, prioritizing your well-being, and carving out space for yourself doesn't mean you're neglecting anyone else. If anything, it makes you better equipped to handle everything life throws your way.

I've had to cut through a lot of noise to figure out what works for me. And if you've ever felt as if you're drowning in advice or trying to do it all – you're not alone. In a world that keeps pushing us to do more, be more, and look perfect while we're at it – I just wanted to create something that feels honest and grounding.

And so this book is for anyone who has ever felt overwhelmed by the surplus of wellness advice out there. The internet can feel like an information minefield – you search for answers and end up with more questions. It's for those who want to take that first step but don't know where to begin. It's for the multitasking moms, the young professionals, and all women in between who just want to feel good in their skin.

I don't have all the answers, but I can promise you this – if I can make peace with my body, mind, and soul, so can you. Health isn't about chasing youth. It's about loving the version of yourself you are today. It's about celebrating the laugh lines, the stretch marks, and everything else that tells the story of your life.

So let's get started. I hope by the end of this book, you realize just how easy it is to be healthy!

PART I

BEAUTY

1
Skin: Glow from the Inside Out

I always say that your skin is a reflection of how you live your life. It tells stories – of late nights, unforgettable vacations, heartbreaks, and the strength that gets you through it all. For me, skincare isn't about vanity. It's self-love in its most tangible form, a way to honour the incredible resilience of our bodies.

People often ask me how I maintain my skin. And while I'd love to share a single magic product, the truth is, it's a mix of rituals, habits, and the occasional indulgence. It's about consistency and listening to what my skin needs – something I wasn't always good at.

In my twenties, skincare meant washing my face and hoping for the best. That changed one morning after a long shoot when my mom handed me a bowl of *besan ubtan* and said, 'Your skin is asking for help.' That was the start of my real skincare journey, and to this day, ubtans are a weekly ritual.

Another memory that stays with me is my mom applying almond oil to her face every evening. I laughed at the shine then, but today, it's my secret weapon too.

Looking back, those early moments — where the ingredients were simple, homemade, and often underestimated — were the real beginnings of my skincare journey.

The Early Days: From Soap to Serums

My skincare journey didn't exactly start with serums and fancy moisturizers. In my twenties, it was as basic as it gets — Margo soap, baby oil, or coconut oil to remove makeup, and zero awareness of sunscreen or moisturizer. My mom and grandmother were my first skincare mentors, but at the time, I didn't fully grasp the value of their wisdom.

Mom would hand me a bowl of ubtan, made out of chickpea flour or besan, turmeric, and almond oil, and say, 'This will nourish your skin.' My grandmother showed me her *nuskhe*, how to massage coconut oil into my face in slow, upward strokes. I'd often roll my eyes, but those simple, natural remedies were quietly laying the foundation for my skincare philosophy.

Back then, skincare wasn't about trends or Instagram-worthy routines. It was about practicality and tradition. I remember watching my mom use sandalwood paste on her face or slice up a tomato to soothe sunburns. While I didn't fully appreciate it at the time, those rituals have become a comforting thread in my life – connecting me to the women who raised me and the simple power of natural care.

How Skin Changes with Age

Ladies, let me be real with you: your skin in your twenties will not be your skin in your forties – and that's OK. The key is to adapt and embrace these changes rather than to resist them.

In my thirties, late nights began announcing themselves under my eyes, and my once-bouncy skin started feeling less forgiving. Hormonal shifts, stress, and a packed schedule all played their part. I leaned on tried-and-tested remedies like aloe vera to soothe and moisturize, while adding vitamin C serums to my routine for a much-needed glow boost.

Pregnancy brought its own challenges – stretch marks, pigmentation, and dullness. Postpartum, I stood in front of the mirror, staring at the uneven patches on my belly, and thinking, 'This doesn't feel like me.' But instead of resenting these changes, I learned to honour them. I used warm almond oil mixed with a few drops of rosehip oil to massage my belly every night. Over time, the stretch marks softened, and so did my view of them. They weren't imperfections; they were proof of everything my body had endured and created.

By my forties, perimenopause introduced new battles – persistent dryness, pigmentation, and that 'tight' feeling no moisturizer seemed to fix. It meant upgrading my skincare game yet again, adding richer creams, retinols, and more powerful serums. But I also leaned deeper into what had always worked: ubtans, aloe vera, and hydration.

The lesson I've learned through every phase? Your skin doesn't ask for perfection – it asks for care, patience, and the willingness to adapt. Every line, spot, or scar tells a story, and I've learned to see them as markers of my resilience rather than as flaws.

My Skincare Routine and Its Evolution

Skincare, for me, is deeply personal – almost as unique as a fingerprint. Over the years, I've tried it all, from whipping up homemade malai and face packs in my kitchen to diving into advanced serums and treatments. But if there's one thing I've learned, it's this: consistency beats everything else.

My mom and grandmother taught me early on that skincare isn't just about the products – it's as much about the ritual as it is about the outcome. It's about taking that moment for yourself, grounding your mind, and nourishing your body.

Of course, my relationship with skincare has evolved over the years. From a time when one moisturizer was deemed sufficient for the whole body to building AM and PM routines, I, like a lot of us, have come far. As I've grown older, I've learned to listen to my skin and tweak my rituals accordingly. What worked in my twenties – basic cleansing and oils – needed upgrades in my thirties, and then in my forties, my routine is a well-balanced mix of home remedies, serums, and sunscreens.

But that sense of connection to tradition anchors my skincare rituals even today. Whether I'm at home, on a shoot, or travelling, I always find time to stick to my skincare routine.

My Morning Skincare Routine: A Ritual for Radiance

Mornings are sacred to me. They set the tone for my entire day, so I treat them as a time to nourish my skin, body, and mind. It all starts with a few grounding rituals.

Soaking in the Sun and Breathing Deeply

I begin my day by spending 15–20 minutes basking in the early morning sunlight, either in my garden or on the balcony. That soft, golden light feels like a natural recharge for both my skin and my spirit. I pair this with deep breathing – nothing complicated, just a few slow, steady rounds – to help me feel grounded and ready for the day ahead.

Hydration from the Inside Out

Next, I sip on warm lemon water. This isn't just about hydration; it feels like hitting the 'reset' button on my body. Lemon is rich in vitamin C, and this ritual always leaves me feeling lighter and more refreshed. If I have extra time, I follow it with my go-to health shot: turmeric, ginger, amla, lemon, and black pepper – a fiery concoction that wakes up my system and keeps inflammation at bay.

Skincare Steps

Once I'm hydrated, it's time for the real magic. I keep my routine simple but effective.

- **Cleansing:** A gentle cleanser tailored to my combination skin.
- **Vitamin C Serum:** My must-have for brightening and protecting my skin from free radicals.
- **Hyaluronic Acid:** To lock in moisture and keep my skin plump.
- **Moisturizer:** A lightweight formula that hydrates without clogging my pores.

- **Sunscreen:** My ultimate shield. Whether it's sunny, cloudy, or even if I'm indoors all day, sunscreen is non-negotiable. I prefer lightweight formulas and reapply diligently if I'm outdoors for long.

Face Yoga

Before stepping into the hustle of the day, I spend five minutes on face yoga. Lifting my cheeks, massaging my jawline, and smoothing out my forehead are small but incredibly effective actions. Over time, this has become my go-to for a natural, sculpted lift. Once you get into it, you'll be making fish faces in the mirror just like me – I get into the full routine a little later, so stay tuned!

DIY Ice Cubes for Hydration and Depuffing

Some mornings, especially after a late night, I use DIY ice cubes made from cucumber juice, aloe vera, or potato juice. Gliding an ice cube over my face instantly depuffs, tightens, helps with dark circles and pigmentation, and leaves me feeling refreshed.

Sun Awareness

Over the years, I've also learned to respect the sun. In my younger days, I'd spend hours baking at the beach with little thought for the damage it could cause. Now I avoid direct sun exposure during peak hours and never skip sunscreen. That said, sunlight is a major ingredient in my magic potion. More about that later!

My Night Skincare Routine: Wind Down and Glow Up

Evenings are my time to unwind, and my skincare routine is central to that process. After a long day of pollution, makeup, and stress, I give my skin the care it deserves.

Double Cleansing

I swear by the double-cleansing method to remove the day's build-up. I start with an oil-based cleanser or balm to melt away makeup, sunscreen, and grime. Next, I follow up with a gentle water-based cleanser. It's a foolproof way to make sure my skin is squeaky clean but not stripped.

Targeted Treatments

Once my skin is clean, I focus on treatments.
- **Retinol (once a week):** To encourage cell renewal and keep fine lines in check.
- **Niacinamide Serum:** To repair, calm, and strengthen the skin barrier.
- **Hyaluronic Acid:** To deeply hydrate and lock in moisture.

- **Moisturizer:** While I prefer lightweight options, I switch to richer creams in winter or when my skin feels extra dry.

Face Yoga and Massage

A light lymphatic massage and gentle tapping around my eyes reduce puffiness and help me relax before bed. If I'm feeling indulgent, I'll even pull out my gua sha stone for a soothing face massage.

Digestive Health

Gut health is key to good skin, so I drink a warm digestive shot before bed. A mix of cumin, fennel, and ajwain (carom seeds) keeps my gut happy and my skin clear.

Skincare for Every Scenario

Skincare isn't one-size-fits-all. It shifts with the demands of the day, whether I'm travelling, shooting, or simply spending a lazy Sunday at home. Over the years, I've learned to tailor my routine to suit these different scenarios, ensuring my skin gets exactly what it needs.

Travel Days: Surviving the Airplane Moisture Vacuum

Airplane cabins are the ultimate test for your skin – dry, pressurized, and utterly unforgiving. I've learned this the hard way. During one trip to Europe, I forgot my hydrating mist, and by the time I landed, my skin felt like parchment paper. Never again!

Now I never board a flight without a rich, heavy moisturizer and a hydrating mist in my carry-on. Before take-off, I slather on moisturizer as if I'm prepping for battle. Lip balm is another must – I can't stress this enough. And makeup? A big no. I let my skin breathe and focus on hydration instead.

For long-haul flights, I also keep a small container of almond oil with me. A quick dab under the eyes mid-flight keeps my skin feeling fresh. It's a small effort, but it makes all the difference when you're stepping off the plane, looking like you just woke up from a nap instead of a long-haul survival mission.

Shoot Days: Battling the Lights, Heat, and Dust

Shoot days are intense – bright lights, long hours, and layers of makeup. In my early days, I didn't realize how much of a toll this took on my skin. During one of my first song shoots, my skin felt like it was on fire by the end of the day.

These days, I prep like a pro. My morning routine starts with a thicker layer of sunscreen – non-negotiable when you're spending hours under hot lights. Between takes, I dab on a hydrating serum or spritz rose water for a quick refresh. During a shoot for 'Chaiyya Chaiyya', the relentless dust and heat were unbearable, so I'd sneak off during breaks to splash water on my face. Sometimes, the simplest tricks work best.

I even take a little bit of DIY skincare to the sets. During a shoot, I once used a turmeric-infused serum I'd made at home. The crew joked that I was 'bringing homemade beauty to Bollywood', but hey, it worked! My skin stayed calm and glowing through the chaos.

Rest Days: Letting Your Skin Breathe

Rest days are my skin's favourite. This is when I completely ditch makeup and focus on deep nourishment. My go-to ritual is a long facial massage with almond or coconut oil. There's something incredibly soothing about massaging your skin while binge-watching your favourite series or reading a good book.

These moments feel luxurious, but they're also therapeutic. I can feel my skin soaking in the nourishment, and I love the natural glow that follows. Sometimes I'll add a turmeric or sandalwood paste for an extra treat.

Regular Days: The Power of Consistency

My regular skincare routine is straightforward: cleanse, treat, moisturize, and protect. It's not flashy or overly complicated, but consistency is the magic ingredient.

I always say skincare isn't about the big, show-stopping rituals – it's about the small, consistent efforts that stack up over time. Those daily moments of care and attention are what build that long-term glow.

Every day brings its own challenges, but with a little care and preparation, your skin can thrive no matter what you're facing.

Skincare Beyond the Face

Skincare isn't just about your face – it's a head-to-toe ritual that nurtures the largest organ of your body. I've always believed that every inch of your skin deserves the same love and attention. Over the years, I've incorporated simple, effective practices to ensure that my body feels as radiant and cared for as my face.

Bath and Shower Rituals: A Daily Spa Moment

My mornings always begin with a warm shower that ends in a quick cold rinse. This simple switch in water temperature tightens the skin, improves circulation, and leaves me feeling invigorated. On days when I want to add a little luxury to my routine, I mix a few drops of almond or coconut oil into my body wash for extra nourishment.

Exfoliation is a cornerstone of my shower routine. On weekends, I turn to my mom's tried-and-tested recipe:

besan mixed with dahi and a pinch of turmeric. This homemade scrub gently removes dead skin cells, leaving my skin soft and glowing. When I'm in the mood for something richer, I whip up a honey and olive oil blend and massage it into my arms and legs before showering. Honey acts as a humectant, drawing moisture into the skin, while olive oil provides deep hydration.

For an indulgent spa-like experience, I sometimes prepare a homemade coffee and sugar scrub. It's excellent for exfoliating. The combination of sugar and coffee stimulates circulation, encourages cell turnover, and leaves the skin incredibly smooth. The caffeine even helps to tighten the skin temporarily, making it a favourite before events or shoots for smooth and healthy-looking skin.

Pigmentation: Natural Solutions for Even-Toned Skin

Pigmentation, especially on elbows, knees, and the neck, has always been a concern for me. Over the years, I've discovered that natural remedies work wonders for evening out these areas.

My favourite solution is a lemon juice and honey paste. The lemon brightens, while honey soothes and prevents irritation. I apply this twice a week, always following up with a rich moisturizer to keep the skin hydrated.

Another recipe I swear by is a rice flour and milk scrub. This combination gently exfoliates while gradually lightening dark patches. It's a slow process, but the results are worth the time taken.

Dry Brushing: A Game Changer for Skin Texture

Dry brushing has become one of my favourite rituals – it's simple, effective, and incredibly satisfying. Using a natural-bristle brush, I make gentle, upward strokes towards the heart before showering. Not only does this promote lymphatic drainage and improve circulation but it also boosts cell turnover, leaving my skin softer and smoother. Over time, I've noticed a visible reduction in the appearance of cellulite and an overall improvement in skin texture.

Making Whole Body Skincare a Ritual

These rituals are essentially moments of self-care that remind me to slow down and connect with my body. Whether it's massaging oil into my stretch marks, exfoliating with homemade scrubs, or simply savouring the sensation of smooth skin after dry brushing, these practices are as much about mindfulness as they are about skincare. My almond and rosehip oil blend, the one I started using postpartum, is still a staple in my routine – it's like a love letter to my skin.

Every body has a story, and every stretch mark, pigment patch, or dry patch is part of that narrative. With a little care, these stories can shine beautifully.

Yoga for Glowing Skin

Yoga isn't just about flexibility or fitness – it's a transformative practice that touches every part of your life, including your skin. When I'm consistent with my yoga practice, my skin thanks me in ways no serum or cream ever could. Fewer breakouts, an even tone, and a glow that feels like it comes from deep within – it's truly my secret weapon.

The beauty of yoga lies in its ability to boost circulation, detoxify the body, and calm inflammation – three things that show up almost instantly on your face. Of course, yoga is a huge part of my overall wellness journey, and I go much deeper into that in the 'Fitness' chapter. So if you're curious about my full practice, asanas, and routines – don't skip that section!

But since we're talking skin, let's start here.

> ### Yoga Poses I Swear By
> Here are my go-to yoga asanas for glowing skin. These poses not only rejuvenate your complexion but also leave your body feeling energized and refreshed.

- **Sarvangasana (Shoulder Stand):** Often called the queen of asanas, this pose works wonders for your skin. Holding it for 3–5 minutes helps flush out toxins, boosts circulation, and gives your face a natural lift.
- **Halasana (Plough Pose):** My ultimate stress-buster. After long days on set, I turn to this to ease fatigue and flood my skin with oxygen. The result? That unmistakable post-yoga glow.
- **Bhujangasana (Cobra Pose):** This powerful pose opens the chest, stretches the skin, and delivers an instant shot of oxygen to the body and face. I swear by it on dull-skin days.
- **Matsyasana (Fish Pose):** A great pose for the throat and jawline, it helps balance hormones and gives your skin a visibly lifted look.
- **Adho Mukha Svanasana (Downward Dog):** A classic that never fails. It boosts blood flow to the face, clears toxins, and leaves you feeling refreshed inside and out.

I make time for at least 20 minutes of these asanas every day, along with pranayama. Deep breathing floods your system with oxygen, calms inflammation, and is one of the simplest, most powerful ways to radiate beauty from within.

Face Yoga: A Workout for Your Skin

I don't stop at full-body yoga – I've also discovered the magic of face yoga: a workout for your facial muscles that tones, lifts, and boosts blood flow, all without a single needle or gadget. It might sound unconventional to some, but now it's part of my daily routine. Whether it's a cheek lift in the mirror or a jawline massage during a phone call, these mini rituals are quick, effective, and surprisingly fun.

> ## My Favourite Face Yoga Moves
>
> - **Forehead Lift:** Place your fingers above your eyebrows and gently push upward, holding for 1–2 minutes. It smooths out fine lines and gives your forehead a relaxed, youthful look.
> - **Jawline Sculpting:** Tilt your head back slightly and use your knuckles to massage along your jawline in upward strokes. It's perfect for tightening the jaw and reducing puffiness.

- **Cheek Lift:** Using three fingers on each cheek, lift the skin upward and hold for 30 seconds. Repeat five times for naturally sculpted cheekbones.
- **Neck Stretch and Tap:** Stretch your neck side to side and lightly tap under your chin to improve circulation and tighten the skin. Simple, but incredibly effective.
- **Balloon Puff or Piano Tap:** Puff your cheeks like a balloon, then gently tap your face with your fingertips like you're playing piano. It boosts collagen, wakes up the skin, and honestly? I'd pick this over the overhyped ice bath any day.

To avoid wrinkles caused by pillow lines, I also make a conscious effort to sleep on my back. It's a small change, but over time, it can make a big difference in keeping your skin smooth.

Gua Sha and Ice Baths: My Skin Saviours

Some mornings, especially after late nights, I need a little extra help. That's where gua sha and ice baths for the face come in.

- **Gua sha:** This smooth jade or rose quartz tool is a game changer. Applying a few drops of

facial oil, I gently glide the tool upward along my cheeks, jawline, and forehead. It helps with lymphatic drainage, reduces puffiness, and feels like a mini spa session at home.
- Ice Baths for the Face (Sort Of): I know dunking your face in ice water is all the rage – it's supposed to tighten pores, reduce puffiness, and give you that fresh, wide-awake look. And while it sounds amazing in theory, I have acute sinusitis, so I steer clear. That said, I've seen it work wonders for people I know. If it's your cup of tea, go for it – but check in with yourself first. It needs a bit of breath control and comfort with cold, so do it only if it *feels* good for you. I'm not an expert, but I've found other ways to get that glow, like the face yoga poses, without freezing my face off!

Hydration: The Underrated Glow Hack

I know, I know – every celebrity ever has credited their glow to 'just drinking water', so I get the scepticism. But trust me, hydration isn't overhyped. If your gut's off, your skin shows it. Beauty doesn't work in a vacuum – it starts from within. Hydration is the simplest, most effective way to care for your skin – but there's a catch. Just drinking litres of plain water won't magically erase dark circles or breakouts overnight. It's about *how* you hydrate.

For me, infused water is a daily ritual that makes hydration fun and effective. Here are some of my favourite combos:

- **Mint, cucumber, and lemon:** Cooling, detoxifying, and refreshing.
- **Orange and basil:** Zesty and energizing.
- **Ginger and lemon:** A spicy twist for extra warmth and detoxification.

When I'm on the go – whether at a shoot or travelling – I carry a bottle of infused water with me. It keeps my skin hydrated and fresh, especially under harsh studio lights or during long flights.

But don't overdo it. I've made the mistake of guzzling too much water, thinking more is better. Spoiler alert: it's not. Over-hydration can lead to puffiness, which is the opposite of what we're going for. I stick to around 2–3 litres a day – just enough to stay hydrated without feeling waterlogged.

Health Shots and Drinks for Glowing Skin

If you ask me, glowing skin starts in the kitchen. No amount of expensive creams can replicate the radiance that comes from nourishing your body from the inside out. That's where my beloved health shots and nutrient-packed drinks come in. They're tiny but mighty, packed with skin-loving ingredients that fight inflammation, boost collagen, and brighten your complexion. Over time, these have become an essential part of my daily routine – and yes, they make a noticeable difference.

Morning Ritual: The Glow Shot

My mornings are incomplete without my turmeric and ginger shot, a true powerhouse for the skin. It's an anti-inflammatory elixir that not only soothes your system but also gives your skin that extra oomph. Here's my simple recipe:

Ingredients
- 1 tsp fresh turmeric (or ½ tsp turmeric powder)
- ½ inch grated ginger
- A pinch of black pepper
- 1 tsp honey
- 1 tbsp warm water

Method
- Mix all the ingredients together and drink it first thing in the morning.

This shot does wonders for reducing redness, boosting circulation, and prepping your skin for the day ahead. And yes, if I skip it for even a few days, my skin notices – I look duller and less refreshed.

Evening Detox: Jeera Pani

My evenings are all about digestion, which plays a critical role in how your skin looks. Enter my family recipe for jeera pani, a soothing and detoxifying drink that I swear by.

Ingredients
- 1 tsp jeera (cumin seeds)
- ½ tsp saunf (fennel seeds)
- ¼ tsp ajwain (carom seeds)
- 2 cups water

Method
- Soak the ingredients for approximately four hours.
- Boil the water for 5–7 minutes until it reduces slightly.
- Strain and sip it warm.

This drink helps with bloating, reduces inflammation, and keeps my skin calm and clear. On days when I'm feeling adventurous, I'll add a squeeze of lemon for an extra detoxifying boost.

Aloe Vera and Wheatgrass Shots

For those late evenings when I want something lighter, I turn to aloe vera or wheatgrass shots. These are incredible for hydration and detoxification, and they're perfect for calming any irritation or redness in the skin. Aloe vera soothes and hydrates the skin. Wheatgrass is packed with antioxidants; it detoxifies and brightens the complexion.

Ubtans and Face Packs: Pantry Secrets for Glowing Skin

I've always believed that you don't need a fancy jar or a trip to an expensive clinic to achieve glowing skin. Some of the best skincare magic happens right in your kitchen. And ubtans and homemade face packs have been a cornerstone of my beauty routine for as long as I can remember.

I grew up watching my mom mix fragrant powders with milk or rose water, transforming simple ingredients into something extraordinary.

All these years later, I find myself doing the same – though I'll admit, I'm often multitasking with a face pack on while prepping for the day!

There's something so satisfying about using natural ingredients. They're gentle, effective, and you know exactly what's going onto your skin – no harsh chemicals, just pure goodness. Plus, there's a certain nostalgia to it. It feels like I'm carrying forward a tradition, one bowl of fragrant powder at a time.

Why Ubtans Work

Ubtans are more than just face packs – they're multitaskers. They cleanse, exfoliate, brighten, and nourish all in one go. The ingredients are simple but powerful. For instance, turmeric fights inflammation, and sandalwood has calming properties.

When I apply an ubtan, it's not just about the glow it gives me. It's a moment to slow down, breathe, and connect with myself.

My Two Go-To Recipes

These are the recipes I return to time and time again. Whether it's before a shoot or on a quiet self-care Sunday, they never fail to leave my skin looking like I've just stepped out of a spa.

Almond and Rose Glow Ubtan

Whenever my skin looks dull or tired, this is my go-to. Almonds provide gentle exfoliation, rose petals calm and brighten, and turmeric adds an antiseptic touch.

Ingredients
- 2 tbsp ground almonds
- 1 tbsp dried rose petals (crushed)
- 1 tsp sandalwood powder
- A pinch of turmeric
- Milk or rose water (to form a paste)

Method
- Mix all the dry ingredients in a bowl.
- Slowly add milk or rose water until you get a thick, spreadable paste.
- Apply evenly over your face and neck, avoiding the eye area.
- Let it dry for 15–20 minutes.
- Once dry, scrub it off in circular motions with lukewarm water.
- Pat your skin dry and follow up with a light moisturizer.

The result is baby-soft skin with an instant glow. I use this once a week, especially before important events or shoots, and it never disappoints.

Hydrating Honey and Oatmeal Face Pack

On days when my skin feels parched, this face pack is my saviour. Honey locks in moisture, oatmeal soothes, and yogurt provides a creamy texture that feels indulgent.

Ingredients
- 2 tbsp oats (finely ground)
- 1 tbsp raw honey
- 1 tbsp yogurt (for extra hydration)
- A few drops of rose water

Method
- Combine the oats, honey, and yogurt in a bowl.
- Add rose water until the consistency is just right – not too thick or runny.
- Apply generously to your face and neck.
- Let it sit for 20 minutes (perfect for a quick meditation).
- Rinse with lukewarm water, gently massaging to exfoliate.

I often use this the night before a big day or after a long flight and end up with plump, hydrated skin that feels like it's had a tall drink of water.

These little recipes are proof that skincare doesn't have to break the bank. Sometimes all you need is a peek into your pantry and a few quiet minutes to yourself.

Makeup and Skin: The Myths and Musts

Let's clear up a common misconception: makeup doesn't ruin your skin – neglecting proper removal does. Over the years, I've learned that how you treat your skin after makeup is just as important as the products you use.

Prepping Your Skin for Makeup

Healthy skin is the best canvas. Before applying makeup, I always prep my skin:
1. Hydrate with a lightweight moisturizer to prevent the makeup from drying out the skin.
2. Sunscreen is a must – it protects from harmful UV rays that can penetrate even through makeup.
3. Use a primer for a smooth base and to extend the wear of your makeup.

The 'Less Is More' Philosophy

When it comes to applying makeup, I'm a firm believer in the 'less is more' approach. Start with the basics – enhance one feature, whether it's your eyes, lips, or cheekbones – and build as needed. Overloading your skin with layers of products can suffocate it, leading to clogged pores and breakouts.

Here's my personal hack: know your skin type and tone. Picking the right shades and formulations makes all the difference. And remember, makeup isn't about hiding – it's about highlighting.

The Non-Negotiable Rule: Removing Makeup

Sleeping with makeup on? That's skincare sabotage. The truth is, makeup left overnight clogs pores, irritates skin, and even accelerates ageing. That's why I never skip double cleansing, especially with waterproof products.

If I've had a particularly long day, I'll indulge in a quick facial massage while cleansing. It's not just about removing makeup – it's about resetting and giving your skin a moment of care.

Brush Hygiene Matters

Let's talk about tools – your makeup brushes. Think of them like your toothbrush – you wouldn't go days without cleaning that, right? Dirty brushes harbour bacteria, which can lead to breakouts and irritation. I clean mine daily with a gentle soap or cleanser. It's a small step that makes a massive difference.

Makeup is fun, transformative, and empowering, but it should always work *with* your skincare routine – not against it. Balance, care, and proper habits ensure your skin stays glowing, with or without makeup.

The Importance of a Good Dermatologist

I love my kitchen rituals, but there's no denying it – sometimes you need a professional. A good dermatologist is like a skincare coach, guiding you through your skin's changing needs and challenges. They've helped me manage everything from pigmentation and sensitivity to understanding ageing skin.

One of my dermatologists once told me something I'll never forget:

'Your skin is an investment, not an expense.'

That simple phrase shifted my mindset. Skincare isn't about chasing trends or jumping on every new product hype – it's about long-term care, grounded in what works for your unique skin.

Why Regular Visits Matter

Even when my skin feels fine, I make it a point to see my dermatologist regularly. Why? Prevention is key. They've taught me the power of:

- **Retinoids:** For cell renewal and anti-ageing.
- **Managing Pigmentation:** Identifying triggers and treating spots effectively.
- **Choosing the Right Sunscreen:** Tailored to my skin type and lifestyle.

There's also a trust factor. When you've got a professional who knows your skin inside out, you can skip the trial-and-error phase and go straight to solutions that work.

When to Call in the Experts

Let's be real — honey and turmeric can't fix everything. If you're dealing with persistent acne, sudden sensitivity, stubborn dry patches, or unexplained rashes, that's your cue to book an appointment!

I once had dry patches that no amount of moisturizer could fix. Turns out, I was deficient in key vitamins. A quick blood test, supplements, and some targeted treatments later, my skin was back on track.

Dermatologists can spot what you might miss – whether it's hormonal imbalances, eczema, or even internal health issues manifesting on your skin.

The best skincare routine is a blend of the traditional and the professional. Trust your dermatologist as much as you trust your pantry remedies, and you'll have a winning combination that keeps your skin glowing for the long haul.

Invasive vs Non-Invasive Treatments

Balance is everything. While I adore my natural remedies and daily skincare rituals, I also appreciate what modern technology can offer – when used mindfully.

Non-Invasive Treatments: Small Wins, Big Results

I'm a fan of non-invasive options like light therapy facials and microdermabrasion. These are great for boosting circulation, refining skin texture, and giving you that extra glow when you need it.

I vividly remember my first light therapy facial; it was before an awards show. My skin was glowing for days – like it had been lit from within.

Invasive Treatments: Proceed with Caution

Now let's talk about the big guns – Botox, fillers, and laser treatments. I'm not against them, but here's the thing: they should enhance, not alter. Moderation is key.

I've seen friends experience amazing results, but I've also witnessed horror stories. A friend once went a little too far with Botox and couldn't smile properly for weeks. That's why I always say:

- **Do your research.** Find a trusted professional.
- **Start small.** Less is more when it comes to invasive treatments.
- **Listen to your skin.** Don't do it just because it's trendy.

The Long Game

Invasive or non-invasive, treatments should always complement your daily habits. No laser or filler can replace good sunscreen, hydration, and cleansing. Skincare isn't a quick fix – it's a lifestyle.

Whether it's a light therapy facial or a rose water spritz, I believe in using every tool at your disposal thoughtfully. Balance and consistency are the real secrets to radiant, healthy skin.

Diet and Skin: What to Eat and What to Avoid

Your skin truly reflects what you eat. Over the years, I've come to realize that it's not just about what you apply on your skin – it's about what you feed it from within. Whenever I indulge in greasy snacks or sugar-loaded desserts, my skin retaliates with dullness or breakouts. But when I nourish my body with the right foods, the glow is undeniable.

Here's my go-to list of skin-loving foods:
1. **Leafy Greens:** Packed with antioxidants that combat free radicals and keep your skin youthful.
2. **Berries and Citrus Fruits:** Rich in vitamin C, they brighten the skin and boost collagen production.
3. **Nuts and Seeds:** Almonds, walnuts, and chia seeds are my favourites. They're full of omega-3s and vitamin E, which keep the skin plump and hydrated.
4. **Turmeric and Ginger:** Anti-inflammatory powerhouses that calm the skin and prevent flare-ups.
5. **Hydrating Foods:** Think cucumbers and watermelons. They work from the inside out to keep your skin moisturized.

It's just as important to know what to skip.
1. **Excess Sugar:** Spikes in sugar levels can lead to inflammation and breakouts.
2. **Fried and Greasy Foods:** These can clog pores and leave your skin looking dull.
3. **Artificial Additives:** Preservatives and chemicals in processed foods can wreak havoc on sensitive skin.

4. **Dairy (in excess):** While some can tolerate it, for many, dairy can lead to breakouts or flare-ups.

The key is balance – listen to your body and adjust your diet accordingly.

Listening to Your Skin

Skincare is deeply personal, and no one knows your skin better than you. The best thing you can do is listen to what it's trying to tell you.

Understanding Trends vs Needs

In today's world of viral skincare hacks, it's easy to get overwhelmed. I've tried my share of trending tips – some amazing, some disastrous. What I've learned is this: just because something works for someone else doesn't mean it will work for you.

Before hopping on a trend, ask yourself:
- Does my skin actually need this?
- Am I addressing a real issue or am I just curious?

Introduce one new product or habit at a time. Your skin needs time to adjust, and if something doesn't work, dial it back.

Sunday Skin Check Ritual

Here's a little habit I swear by: a weekly 'skin check' every Sunday night.

- Stand in front of the mirror and cleanse your face.
- Look closely for signs of tightness, dullness, or redness.
- Adjust your routine for the upcoming week based on what you see.

Your skin changes with the weather, diet, stress, and so much more. Being attuned to these shifts helps you stay ahead of any issues and tweak your skincare as needed.

Skincare isn't about perfection – it's about understanding and nurturing your skin as it evolves. Listening to your skin and responding with care is the best beauty hack you'll ever need.

Final Word: Skincare as Self-Love

From health shots to face yoga, these rituals aren't just skin-deep – they help me feel grounded and clear from the inside out. They're not about trends or expensive fixes, but about tuning in, staying consistent, and using simple tools like breath, movement, and hydration. Over time, it's these small, steady habits – not the flashy treatments — that make the biggest difference. The proof, as they say, is in the pudding.

Skincare is more than just routines or products — it's a celebration of self-care. At the end of the day, your skincare should feel like a moment of self-love, not a burdensome checklist. Whether it's a DIY face pack made with pantry staples or the glow from a trusted serum, it's about finding what makes you feel good. Embrace your skin as it is — flaws, changes, and all. Your skin is always communicating — listen to it, nurture it, and remember, a happy you equals glowing skin. When you treat your skin with kindness, it reflects your care back to you. Your skincare journey is as unique as you are — cherish it and make it a joyful ritual.

2
Hair: The Crown You Never Take Off

Hair – our crowning glory, right? It's often one of the first things people notice about us, but it's also a reflection of how well we take care of ourselves. I see my hair as more than just a style statement. It's a reflection of my experiences, of how much I've learned (and sometimes, of how much I've suffered through trial and error) when it comes to looking after it.

Let's be real – hair is a tricky thing. It's not just about genetics; it's about the life you lead, how much TLC you give it, and yes, sometimes about how much damage you put it through. From my younger years, where I didn't think twice about the countless hairstyles and products I tried, to now, where I've finally found a rhythm, my hair journey has been an evolution. But here's what I've learned: no matter how much you change, your hair always needs care, attention, and a little bit of love.

Hair Through the Decades and Beyond

Hair is always changing, just like we are. From the carefree days of our twenties to the more thoughtful care in our thirties and forties, our hair goes through its own transformations.

The Twenties: A Time of Youthful Glow

In your twenties, your hair is often at its most vibrant. Your follicles are working at full capacity, and your scalp is relatively healthy, which means thicker, stronger strands. Generally at this point, you don't need to worry too much about hair loss or thinning – it's all about experimenting with different styles, colours, and textures.

In my twenties, my hair was thick and glossy. Of course I still had the occasional bad hair day, but I could put it through anything – constant styling, colouring – and it bounced right back. It's that period of life when you're confident in your hair's natural beauty and when everything seems to come easy.

But even in our twenties, it's important to start laying the foundation for hair care. Yes, you can enjoy the fun and freedom of styling, but it's the perfect time to start adopting healthy habits, like oil massages and hydrating shampoos. You don't need heavy-duty treatments, but keeping things simple and nurturing will pay off in the long run.

The Thirties: The First Signs of Change

As you move into your thirties, the changes in your body start to show, and your hair is no exception. Many women start noticing thinning or more breakage as their hair begins to lose some of that volume and elasticity. This is when the first signs of ageing begin to appear – don't panic! Your hair might start feeling a little more fragile or less bouncy, and that's completely normal.

Hormonal changes are a key factor here. Your hormones fluctuate due to stress, lifestyle, or just the natural ageing process, and these shifts can lead to more hair fall. Additionally, pregnancy and the postpartum period (which can often occur in your thirties) can wreak havoc on your hair's texture and volume.

I definitely noticed the change in my thirties – suddenly, my hair wasn't as thick as it once was. Even my stylist pointed out that I wasn't getting the same volume from my roots. It was a humbling realization, but I adapted, incorporating deeper conditioning treatments and stronger protein-based masks to maintain my hair's strength and texture.

The Forties: The Slowdown Begins

When you hit your forties, you may notice more pronounced hair thinning, especially around the crown. It's also common for hair to lose its natural lustre and start feeling drier and more brittle. The ageing process continues, and this is when perimenopause starts affecting many women. Along with other changes in your body, you may notice that your hair isn't as thick or strong as it once was, and grey strands may start appearing more frequently.

I found that I needed to be much more mindful about my hair care routine. This is when I started focusing on hydration and nourishment, using oils and masks more regularly. Vitamins and supplements became part of my daily routine too, with an emphasis on collagen. You can't expect your hair to stay the same with age, but with a little effort, it can still look fabulous.

Pregnancy and Postpartum: The Roller Coaster Ride

During pregnancy many women notice their hair is fuller and shinier. The surge in hormones can make your hair thicker and more voluminous, which is why some pregnant women enjoy a 'glowing' hair period. Unfortunately, once the baby is born and the hormonal shifts settle down, it's common to experience postpartum hair loss. This can come as a shock, especially after enjoying the pregnancy glow.

During my pregnancy, I noticed my hair grew thicker. But once I delivered, I began losing handfuls of hair! It was scary, but I knew it was temporary. After giving birth, it took a few months to get back to my usual routine. I focused on gentle products and made sure I was getting enough nutrients to aid the recovery process.

Perimenopause and Menopause: The Transition

Perimenopause and menopause mark a period where hair texture can change significantly. During perimenopause, our bodies go through a series of hormonal changes that can lead to increased hair shedding, dryness, and thinner strands. The loss of estrogen (the female hormone), combined with the increase in androgens (male hormones), can shrink hair follicles, resulting in finer, thinner hair.

In my forties, I began experiencing this first-hand, and I noticed that my hair wasn't holding the same shape it once did. It wasn't as bouncy, and the volume I was used to was decreasing. At this stage you must adjust your hair care routine to account for the changes. Moisturizing shampoos, hydrating oils, and gentle styling routines became more important to me.

With the right care, it's possible to embrace the changes. And while our hair may not stay as youthful and thick as it once was, it's about finding what works best for you at every stage of life and ensuring you still feel confident and fabulous.

Covid-19 and Hair: A Global Struggle

The Covid-19 pandemic took a toll on my hair in more ways than one. It wasn't just the stress but the isolation, poor nutrition, disrupted routines, and overall strain on my body. I noticed more shedding than ever before, and it was as if my hair was reflecting everything I was going through inside.

And I know I wasn't alone. So many people experienced unexpected hair fall during this time. Stress, sleep disturbances, and poor food habits all contributed. It was frustrating, even emotional, at times. But once I began focusing on getting my health back on track – eating better, staying hydrated, adding supplements like collagen – things gradually improved.

That phase reminded me of something I now deeply believe: your hair doesn't lie. It mirrors your internal well-being. When you feel good on the inside, it shows up on the outside too. With time, patience, and care, my hair began to bounce back, just like the rest of me.

My Hair Care Regimen

When it comes to hair care, my regimen is all about balance – incorporating the right oils, gentle cleansing, and nourishing conditioners to keep my hair healthy, hydrated, and strong.

Oiling: The Ancient Ritual

I grew up with one clear rule: oiling was non-negotiable. Every week, my mother would sit me down for a champi (head massage), slathering my hair with nourishing oils – sometimes coconut, sometimes almond. It wasn't just a beauty treatment; it was bonding time, a ritual of relaxation and recharging. Even today, I find it incredible how this age-old practice remains one of the most effective ways to nourish hair from the roots.

In my twenties, I brushed off oiling as something my mother did. My hair was thick, my scalp low-maintenance, and I was carefree. But as I grew older, things changed – my hair became thinner, more brittle, and clearly in need of more attention. That's when I began to truly practise what I preach: oiling, but with intention.

Over time, my approach evolved. I used to oil my hair heavily, sometimes leaving it in for 24 hours. But I eventually realized that excessive oiling – and repeated shampooing to get it out – was causing breakage and weakening my strands. Now I oil my hair once every 15 days. It's no longer about how *much* oil I use, but *how* I use it.

A gentle scalp massage with a little oil for 10–15 minutes is more than enough to activate blood circulation and nourish the roots. It's not about loading up the hair but about stimulating the scalp – giving it what it needs without overdoing it.

I've always gravitated towards ayurvedic oils, something my grandmother swore by. Over the years, I've experimented with different blends, but one recipe has stayed with me. It's a treasured family tradition – and here's the secret blend I still make and use:

Homemade Ayurvedic Hair Oil

This oil is packed with ingredients known for their restorative and nourishing properties. My mother and grandmother always made it fresh, and I still do the same today.

Ingredients
- 100 ml coconut oil
- 100 ml olive oil
- 100 ml castor oil
- 1 tbsp methi (fenugreek) seeds

- A handful of fresh curry leaves
- 1 tbsp shoe flower (hibiscus) petals

Method
- In a small pan, heat the oils on a low flame.
- Add the methi seeds and curry leaves. Let them infuse in the oil for 5–10 minutes.
- Once the oil is infused with the herbs, strain and store in a clean bottle.

This oil can be used weekly for a head massage, which helps stimulate the scalp, improve circulation, and promote healthy hair growth.

Cleansing: Gentle yet Effective

Cleansing is where the fun begins – but also where many of us go wrong. For years, I used shampoos with sulphates, thinking that squeaky-clean feeling meant they were doing their job. What I didn't realize was that those harsh chemicals were stripping my hair of its natural oils, leaving it dry and brittle.

Now I choose sulphate-free shampoos that are gentler on the scalp yet effective at removing build-up. I also lean towards ayurvedic shampoos and conditioners made with natural ingredients like shikakai, amla, and neem.

Shikakai, in particular, has been a game changer. It's a gentle cleanser that lathers beautifully and strengthens my hair without drying it out. I grind dried shikakai pods into a fine powder, mix a teaspoon of the powder with water to form a smooth paste, and massage it into my scalp before rinsing. Its natural acidity helps balance the scalp's pH while preserving moisture – leaving my hair soft, shiny, and refreshed.

If you're dealing with heavy product build-up, a simple final rinse can work wonders. Two tablespoons of apple cider vinegar diluted with half a litre of water clears residue and balances the scalp, while a beer rinse adds volume and shine. These quick fixes leave your hair feeling light, clean, and much easier to manage.

Conditioning: Hydrate and Protect

When I was younger, I didn't really understand the importance of conditioning. I'd wash and go, maybe slap on some conditioner when I remembered. But now? It's a ritual I take seriously. When I started seeing hair thinning and breakage, I upped my conditioning game, choosing products that repair and hydrate. In fact, I now swear by deep conditioning. Gone are the days of treating it as an occasional indulgence. My hair needs this extra boost of nourishment every few weeks to maintain its health. After all, it's the age of multi-step routines, and my hair deserves the same care that I give my skin.

My go-to recipe for a natural conditioner? A mix of curd and honey. It sounds simple, but it works wonders. The curd hydrates, while the honey locks in moisture.

Curd and Honey Hair Conditioner

Ingredients
- 2 tbsp plain curd
- 1 tbsp honey
- 1 tbsp olive oil (optional, for extra hydration)

Method
- Mix all the ingredients to form a smooth paste.
- Apply to damp hair, focusing on the ends.
- Leave it on for 15–20 minutes before rinsing with lukewarm water.

Egg and Olive Oil Hair Mask

I also regularly use egg-based hair masks — something I've been doing since childhood.

My mom's tried-and-tested method involved egg whites for protein and yolks for moisture. I also mix in other ingredients like olive oil and honey to create a rich, replenishing mask.

Ingredients
- 1 egg (use the yolk for dry hair, the white for oily hair)
- 1 tbsp olive oil
- 1 tbsp honey

Method
- Beat the egg, then mix in olive oil and honey.
- Apply to damp hair, ensuring it's evenly coated.
- Leave for 20–30 minutes, then rinse with lukewarm water (to avoid cooking the egg!).

These masks leave my hair shiny and soft, providing much-needed hydration, especially after exposure to heat and styling.

Yoga for Healthy Hair

Of course, I have yoga poses up my sleeve for hair too! Beyond fitness and skin, certain poses help increase blood flow to the scalp, nourish the hair follicles, and help promote healthier, stronger hair. It's all about giving your scalp the attention it deserves – along with the rest of your body. I make time for yoga every day, even if it's just for 30 minutes. The poses I swear by are sarvangasana (shoulder stand) and bhujangasana (cobra pose), which stimulate circulation to the scalp and improve the overall health of your hair.

> ## Yoga Poses and Their Benefits for Healthy Hair
> ### Sarvangasana (Shoulder Stand)
> *How to Do It*
> 1. Start by lying on your back and lifting your legs straight up towards the ceiling.
> 2. Lift your hips and back, supporting your weight with your hands placed on your lower back.
> 3. Keep your legs straight and hold this position for 30 seconds to 1 minute.
> 4. Focus on deep breathing – inhale through the nose and exhale through the mouth.
>
> *Benefits*
> - Increases blood circulation to the scalp, promoting healthy hair growth.

- Strengthens the upper body and core.
- Helps improve hormonal balance, which is essential for maintaining healthy hair.
- Reduces stress, which can be a major factor in hair loss.

Bhujangasana (Cobra Pose)

How to Do It

1. Lie flat on your stomach with your palms placed directly under your shoulders.
2. Slowly lift your chest and head off the ground, using your back muscles.
3. Arch your back and raise your chest higher, making sure your elbows are close to your body.
4. Hold the position for 15–30 seconds, breathing deeply throughout.

Benefits

- Opens up the chest, which helps improve oxygen flow throughout the body.
- Helps reduce stress and fatigue, which are often associated with hair thinning.
- Strengthens the spine and improves overall posture.

> Both these poses offer a great way to enhance hair health naturally, by stimulating circulation and reducing stress — all factors that contribute to stronger, shinier hair.

I've found that consistency is key. Ideally, I try to practise these poses every day, but even a few times a week will bring on the benefits. Hold each pose for 30 seconds to 1 minute, and repeat them 2–3 times to get the circulation going. These poses don't need to be performed for long periods, but incorporating them into your daily practice can work wonders over time. Yoga is about listening to your body, and the benefits it brings to your hair are just a bonus along with all the other ways it strengthens your body and mind.

Maintaining Healthy Hair: From Care to Treatment

I wish I could say every day is a good hair day for me — but that's far from the truth. One shoot memory in particular still makes me laugh (no, I'm not telling you which one!). I decided to try something new: sleek, super-straight hair with a sharp middle part. It looked perfect in the mirror, as I myself was feeling — until I stepped onto the beach set. The wind and humidity had other plans. Within 10 minutes, my hair was frizzing in all directions and I had a mildly electrocuted look. We had to stop midway to rework the look, and we eventually went back to my soft waves. Lesson learned: listen to your hair. It knows what it wants, and fighting it rarely ends well.

Healthy hair doesn't happen by accident — it's a mix of regular care, nourishing rituals, and a little help when needed. For me, it starts with the basics: trimming, conditioning, and listening closely to what my hair needs at any given time. Whether it's a quick oil massage before a shower or a deep salon treatment after a stretch of heavy styling, I've learned to read my hair's signals and respond accordingly.

Regular trims are non-negotiable. I try to get a cut every 6–8 weeks — not to switch up the look, but to keep split ends at bay and maintain the hair's strength and bounce. It's a small habit that goes a long way in preventing breakage and keeping things fresh. Between trims, I rely on scalp nourishment and deep hydration. A warm oil massage, sulphate-free shampoo, and moisturizing conditioner are my go-to trio for keeping my strands healthy without stripping away their natural oils.

Of course, there are times when everyday care isn't enough. That's when I lean on professional treatments to give my hair a bit of a reset. When my strands feel dry or lacklustre, a keratin treatment brings back the shine and softness. If I've been using heat tools a little too often, a protein treatment helps rebuild strength and bounce. These aren't frequent indulgences – they're thoughtful interventions when my hair needs a boost.

I've also tried PRP, platelet-rich plasma, for hair thinning and growth. It's not a magic fix, but it *is* a science-backed treatment that has worked for me when my scalp needed extra support. It improves circulation and rejuvenates the hair follicles, helping create a healthier environment for growth. But even so, PRP complements – it doesn't replace – my regular care rituals.

And honestly? Some of my favourite treatments still come straight from my kitchen. A spoonful of curd and honey for deep conditioning, or castor oil and almond oil for hydration and growth – these homemade masks have been part of my routine for years. They may not give you overnight results, but if you stay consistent, they'll work their magic from the inside out.

In the end, hair care is a long-term relationship. It's not about chasing trends or one-off treatments, but about creating a routine that feels right for you. For me, it's that balance – knowing when to stick to the tried-and-tested home rituals and when to reach for professional care. That's what keeps my hair feeling strong, nourished, and full of life.

Bonus Tips for Every Scenario

- **Travel:** Cabin air can be incredibly drying, so I always carry a hydrating hair mist or leave-in conditioner. A wide-toothed comb is another travel essential – it helps detangle without causing breakage.
- **Shoots:** Long hours under harsh lights and constant styling can be tough on the hair. I keep a nourishing serum or light oil in my bag to tame frizz and flyaways. A quick touch-up mid-shoot can make all the difference.
- **Rest Days:** Let your hair breathe. No styling, no heat – just a deep-conditioning mask to restore moisture and revive the texture. Think of it as a mini spa treatment for your strands.
- **Regular Days:** Stick to your basics. Shampoo, conditioner, and oiling – done right and done consistently – are what truly keep your hair strong, shiny, and healthy.

What to Eat and Drink for Healthy Hair

Hair health starts at the roots – and that means paying attention to what's on your plate. I focus on a nutrient-rich diet that supports my scalp, strengthens my strands, and promotes steady growth.

I load up on eggs, almonds, sweet potatoes, and spinach – and when needed, I supplement. These foods have B-vitamins, especially B3 and B6, that are essential for healthy hair. Omega-3 fatty acids from chia seeds, walnuts, and salmon keep my scalp nourished, while vitamin E – found in avocados, leafy greens, and seeds – boosts circulation and supports overall hair vitality.

Soaked almonds and raisins are also my go-to snacks for hair health. Soaked almonds are rich in vitamin E, which promotes healthy hair growth and helps repair damaged hair. Raisins, high in iron and vitamin C, support healthy circulation, which in turn nourishes the hair follicles for stronger, shinier hair. Combined, these ingredients are excellent for both hair and skin health.

Hydration also plays a major role. I begin each day with a turmeric and ginger health shot. It's anti-inflammatory, energizing, and great for circulation. I also love infusing my water with mint, cucumber, and lemon – it's refreshing and supports both hair and skin health.

In the chapter on food, I'll be sharing some of my favourite recipes and go-to ingredients that have become staples in my hair care diet. Beauty really does begin in the kitchen!

Brazil Nut Powder Recipe

One of my favourite natural remedies for supporting healthy hair is a homemade seed mix I swear by. It's packed with selenium, a key mineral for scalp health, along with other nourishing ingredients.

Ingredients
- A handful of roasted Brazil nuts
- 2 tbsp pumpkin seeds
- 1 tbsp chia seeds
- 1 tbsp flaxseeds
- A handful of makhana (fox nuts)
- A handful of walnuts
- A handful of almonds (or soaked almonds)
- Raisins (optional, for added sweetness)

Method
- Dry-roast all the nuts and seeds lightly to release their natural oils.
- Grind them into a fine powder.
- Store in an airtight container.

I mix a tablespoon of this powder with warm water every morning, and it works wonders for boosting hair strength and supporting healthy growth. The result? A light, nourishing drink that supports hair growth and skin elasticity and gives me that enviable 'lit-from-within' glow. It's a simple, nutrient-packed addition to my daily routine.

The Importance of Protein and How Much Is Enough

When it comes to hair health, protein plays a major role. Since our hair is made primarily of keratin – a structural protein – it's essential to have enough protein in your diet to keep your strands strong, resilient, and healthy. Of course, your exact needs will depend on your body weight, lifestyle, and overall health.

But here's something many people miss: more isn't always better. Excessive protein intake can put unnecessary strain on your kidneys, and if your body doesn't use that extra protein, it could be stored as fat. So it's all about balance.

If you're struggling with thinning hair, start by looking at your plate. Include protein-rich foods like lean meats, fish, eggs, beans, and tofu. And if you're vegetarian or vegan, you can still meet your needs with smart plant-based choices – think lentils, chickpeas, quinoa, seeds, and nuts. Getting the right amount of protein consistently can make a visible difference in the strength, density, and texture of your hair.

Supplements for Healthy Hair

While a balanced diet is the foundation of healthy hair, I've found that sometimes your body just needs a little extra support. If you're dealing with thinning, dryness, or sudden shedding, adding a few key supplements can really help.

Collagen

Collagen isn't just great for skin – it's also fantastic for your hair. Collagen helps build keratin, which is the structural protein in hair. As we age, our collagen production decreases, leading to thinner, weaker hair. I include collagen peptides in my daily routine, mixed into my morning drink or smoothie, to support hair health and reduce hair fall. (Of course, it may take a few months to see results – consistency is key.)

Iron and Vitamin D

Iron helps carry oxygen to your hair follicles, and without it, you could experience hair thinning or loss. Many women, particularly during their menstrual years, are prone to iron deficiency, which can directly affect hair health. Similarly, vitamin D plays a crucial role in regulating the hair growth cycle. I ensure I get enough through sunlight or supplements to keep my hair follicles in top shape.

Omega-3 Fatty Acids

These healthy fats help nourish the scalp, keep hair hydrated, and promote growth. I include fish oils and flaxseed oils in my diet, particularly during the colder months, when my scalp tends to feel drier.

Zinc

Zinc is essential for tissue growth and repair, including your hair follicles. It also helps regulate the oil glands around the follicles, preventing dryness and flakiness. I've found that balancing my zinc intake has helped improve my hair's texture and strength.

A Word on Dosage

Supplements can significantly boost your hair health, but it's important not to overdo them. Too much of certain vitamins – like vitamin A or zinc – can have adverse effects, including hair loss. Always consult a doctor or nutritionist before adding new supplements to your routine to ensure they're safe and appropriate for your needs. (What works for me might not work for you – and that's OK!)

The Silent Saboteurs

Maintaining healthy hair is not just about external application of products – it's deeply connected to what's going on inside your body. Stress and nutritional deficiencies often go unnoticed, but they are crucial to your hair's health. It's easy to think a good shampoo or conditioner will suffice, but it's these silent stressors that can have a huge impact on your hair's health and growth cycle.

Stress

Stress can wreak havoc on your body – and your hair is no exception. When you're under pressure, your body releases cortisol, which is great in small bursts but disruptive when it's constantly elevated. Chronic stress can push hair follicles into a resting phase, causing a condition called telogen effluvium, where hair falls out more easily and in greater volume.

I've had my share of stressful periods, especially during intense shoot schedules or personal ups and downs, and I've seen the effects on my hair first-hand. My trichologist helped me understand the connection, and that awareness changed how

I approach stress. If you're noticing sudden or excessive hair loss, stress might be the culprit. Find tools that help you manage it – yoga, meditation, breath work, or even long nature walks – and give your hair a chance to recover from the inside out.

Deficiencies

Your hair is one of the first places where a nutrient deficiency shows up. If your diet is lacking in essentials like iron, vitamin D, vitamin B12, or protein, it can weaken the hair shaft, slow growth, and increase shedding. For example, iron deficiency, especially common among women, is a major reason for hair fall. Vitamin D supports hair follicle cycling, while B12 keeps your scalp and follicles oxygenated and nourished.

That's why I pay close attention to what I eat – and I check in with my doctor regularly. A simple blood test can tell you where your nutrient levels stand and help prevent problems before they show up on your scalp.

If you're noticing changes in your hair – whether it's thinning, breakage, or dullness – look inward first. Start by adding leafy greens, lean proteins, healthy fats, and whole foods to your daily diet. Supplements can help too, but there's no substitute for a balanced, nourishing plate.

When to See an Expert

If you're dealing with severe hair loss, it's essential to consult a dermatologist or trichologist to get to the root cause. Dandruff, dermatitis, and psoriasis are common scalp issues that can cause discomfort and hair thinning, especially in our country's tropical climate. For dandruff, natural remedies like tea tree oil and aloe vera can soothe the scalp, but in more severe cases, please see a doctor who might recommend medicated shampoos or topical treatments, instead of experimenting by yourself.

How Colouring Affects Hair

Colouring and bleaching can be transformative. That first week after a colour appointment is always such a thrill! But while the excitement is real, it's important to remember that hair colour, especially bleach, can also have a lasting impact. I've experimented with everything – from fiery red to cool blonde and ash blonde – and while these shades gave me the look I was after, they didn't come without consequences. Bleaching, in particular, has been a learning curve for me. It strips the hair of moisture, leaving it more porous and prone to breakage. The more you bleach, the more vulnerable your hair becomes, so I've had to become really thoughtful about how I colour my hair.

When I first started colouring my hair, I didn't fully grasp how much impact it would have on my strands. I was too focused on trying new shades to consider the long-term effects. Over time, I noticed my hair feeling drier, thinner, and losing its natural shine. Now, I'm much more careful with the types of colours I go for and how often I refresh them. I've learned that it's not about completely avoiding chemicals, but choosing the right products and ensuring that I hydrate my hair consistently.

I've never been one to hide my age. While I don't have many greys just yet, I don't feel the need to cover them when they do start appearing. Grey hair? If it works, go for it! I'm not in a race to become a Silver Fox – I'm not trying to prove anything to anyone. I colour my hair when I feel like it and leave the rest up to nature.

While I've never really tried pastels or neon shades myself, I can tell you that they're a lot of fun if you're after a bold change. These vibrant hues can really make a statement, but they tend to be harder on your hair than the more natural shades. They often require more maintenance and extra hydration to keep your hair from drying out. If you want to play with colour in a more experimental way, just be prepared for more care, and make sure you're using products that are designed to maintain that vibrancy.

And then there's ammonia. It's found in a lot of hair dyes, and while it's great for opening the hair cuticle and allowing colour to penetrate, it can cause damage. Ammonia strips away moisture and weakens the hair, leading to dryness and breakage. That's why I now opt for ammonia-free dyes whenever I colour my hair – they're gentler on my strands and scalp.

Through all my experiences with hair colour, I've learned that moderation and the right care are key. Healthy hair will always be more important than following trends. It's about finding a balance that works for you and keeping your hair in the best possible condition, whatever colour you choose.

Taming Frizzy Hair

Frizz is something I've definitely had to learn to manage over the years. It can feel like an ongoing battle, but I've figured out how to deal with it by using the right products to keep my hair healthy, hydrated, and smooth, while embracing my natural texture.

Let's clear something up first: frizz isn't always a bad thing. In some cases, it's simply the natural wave or curl in your hair that's trying to break free. For those with naturally wavy or curly hair, what looks like frizz is really just your hair's natural texture coming through. But if you're trying to tame those waves into straightness, that's when things get tricky.

I've had my share of days when frizz was out of control, especially in my younger years when I didn't quite know how to handle it. There was a time I used to straighten my hair every day in an attempt to make it sleek. While straightening gave me that smooth, polished look temporarily, it only weakened my hair and made it more prone to frizz in the long run. I learned that over-styling is often a recipe for more frizz.

Instead, I focus on hydration to keep frizz at bay. Leave-in conditioners are my go-to for smoothing and adding moisture, and a good serum helps lock in hydration and gives my hair that sleek, shiny look. I've found that using a serum that adds weight to the hair without making it greasy works wonders. And when it comes to heat styling, I try to keep it to a minimum, because excessive heat only strips the hair of moisture, making frizz worse.

One of my favourite tricks? A silk pillowcase. It might sound simple, but it really works. Silk causes less friction than cotton, so it reduces tangling and breakage while you sleep. Plus, it helps to keep hair smooth and shiny, even if you have naturally wavy or curly hair. In the end, managing frizz is about knowing your hair and working with it rather than trying to fight against it.

The Perils of Tying Your Hair Too Tight

I love a sleek ponytail as much as the next person. But over the years, I've seen how tight hairstyles can do more harm than good – something both hairstylists and trichologists have warned me about.

- **Traction Alopecia:** If you keep pulling your hair back tightly, over time, it can cause hair loss right from the scalp. It's called traction alopecia, and it's not just a buzzword – it's real, and it can be permanent if ignored.
- **Breakage:** Tight buns and ponytails can strain the strands and cause them to snap.
- **Scalp Tension:** I used to get headaches and only later realized it was from how tight my updos were!

Now, I try to be gentler – using soft hair ties, alternating styles, and letting my scalp breathe in between. Small changes, but they've made a big difference.

Takeaways

- **Know Your Hair Type:** Understanding your hair type is the first step to choosing the right products and care routine.

- **Consistency Is Key:** Regular oiling, cleansing, and conditioning are essential for maintaining healthy, hydrated hair.
- **Hydration:** Moisture is a must! Whether through leave-in conditioners, oils, or deep conditioning treatments, keep your hair hydrated to prevent dryness and damage.
- **Diet and Lifestyle Matter:** A healthy, balanced diet with essential vitamins like omega-3s, and vitamin D is crucial for strong, shiny hair. Don't forget the importance of hydration, sleep, and stress management.
- **Gentle Handling:** Be kind to your hair. Avoid tight hairstyles and excessive heat styling, and always use the right tools to detangle and brush.
- **Age Gracefully:** As your hair changes over the years, adapt your routine to nourish and protect it. Embrace the journey of growing older with grace and healthy hair.

Final Word

Taking care of your hair is a lifelong commitment, but it doesn't need to be complicated. The basics – oil, hydration, a good diet, and consistency – go a long way. Your hair reflects your overall health, so treating it with love and care will always yield the best results. Remember, it's not about following the latest trends or covering up your age; it's about finding what works for you and maintaining healthy, beautiful hair no matter the stage of life. Stick to the fundamentals, trust the process, and your hair will thank you.

3

Magic Potion: Sleep, Water, Sunshine

When it comes to wellness, beauty, and maintaining a balanced life, there are three essentials I always swear by – sleep, water, and sunshine. They're my personal magic potions – the quiet constants behind everything I do to stay healthy, happy, and glowing.

If skincare is where I begin and hair care is how I express myself, then this chapter is about the pillars that support it all. Because no glow serum or conditioning mask can truly work its magic unless the basics are taken care of. We often chase new treatments or trendy fixes, but the real transformation starts with these three elements. They don't just affect how I look – they impact how I feel, my mental clarity, energy levels, and even hormonal balance. Sleep resets the body and mind. Water hydrates from within, bringing that plump, dewy glow no cream can fake. And sunshine? It fuels my spirit and gives my skin the boost it needs – inside and out.

I've come to believe that these aren't just background wellness habits. They're non-negotiables.

And when I treat them as such, everything else – my skin, my hair, my mood – begins to fall into place. Incorporating sleep, water, and sunshine into your daily life isn't about being perfect – it's about making small, conscious choices that support your well-being. These basics create a strong foundation so that everything else you do – whether it's applying a mask or taking a supplement – can actually do its job.

So let these three guide you, the way they guide me. When you invest in them, you're not just chasing beauty or fitness. You're nurturing the core of your health – and that inner glow always finds its way to the surface.

Sleep: The Ultimate Restorative Elixir

Sleep is often underrated, but trust me when I say it's the most important part of my wellness routine. A good night's sleep isn't only about rest – it's when the real magic happens for your body and mind. That's when your body repairs, replenishes, and regenerates. And honestly, who doesn't love waking up feeling fresh and ready to conquer the day.

When you sleep, your body goes into full repair mode. It replenishes cells, regenerates tissue, and balances your hormones. On the flip side, when you're sleep-deprived, stress kicks in. Cortisol levels rise, and your skin starts showing the signs – breakouts, dullness, even dark circles. I've seen it all first-hand. It can become a vicious cycle.

Aiming for seven to nine hours of sleep each night is my golden rule. But it's not only about how long you sleep but also about how well you sleep. Deep sleep is when your body produces the most growth hormone, which helps regenerate skin cells, improve hair texture, and maintain a youthful glow. So it's not only about getting into bed early but about creating a routine that promotes deep, uninterrupted rest.

How to Achieve Good and Deep Sleep

Sleep is one of life's greatest gifts. Seriously. I always say my top three favourite things are water, sunlight, and sleep. These three are the backbone of everything I do to feel good. When I make sure I'm ticking these boxes, everything else falls into place. It's like the perfect trifecta for well-being. But not everyone needs the same amount of sleep. Some people function fine on four hours, others on six. Me? I need a solid eight. If I don't get my sleep, I'm just not the same person.

That said, it's not just about counting the hours. The real magic lies in the quality of sleep. I've learned that all the hours in the world won't make a difference if the sleep isn't deep or uninterrupted. That's why consistency is key. I have created a calming bedtime routine to tell my body it's time to wind down. Dimming the lights, stepping away from screens, and giving myself a moment to just be still. It's like setting the stage for peaceful slumber.

This wasn't always the case. When I was travelling constantly for shoots, bouncing between time zones and running on adrenaline, I learned the hard way how burnout creeps in without quality rest. That's when I realized something important: you have to train your body to unwind – just like you train your body in the gym. It's really about mind over body. And for that, you need consistency.

I know people who suffer from chronic sleep issues. They can get into bed at 10.30 p.m. but won't fall asleep before 2 a.m. – no matter what. So it's not about lying down early but about learning how to switch off. From your phone, from your TV, from stressful thoughts, or late-night arguments. Your body needs cues. Everyone unwinds differently. Some people meditate. Some sip on warm milk. Others swear by a quick bath or a few pages of a book. Some even enjoy a quiet drink at the end of the day. Whatever it is, the point is to find what works for you – and stick with it. You can't try it for two days and say '*arre, hua nahi*'. It's not a quick fix. It's a rhythm you create over time.

That's the only way your body starts to understand when it's time to slow down and truly rest.

The Power of Your Bedtime Routine

I've had my share of late-night shoots, where I'd come home and plop straight into bed, expecting to pass out instantly. Over time, I realized I'd been underestimating how much the little things — like winding down properly — matter in turning sleep from just rest into real recovery. Creating a calming, sleep-friendly environment is an absolute game changer. Here's what I've found helps me get the best sleep:

- **Avoid Caffeine and Stimulants:** I had to learn this the hard way. I used to love my coffee, but I realized it was messing with my sleep, especially after 4 p.m. If you want to hit the pillow and drift off, stay away from caffeine or nicotine four to six hours before bed. I swapped my evening coffee for herbal teas, like chamomile or tulsi, and let me tell you, it made all the difference.
- **Blue Light Exposure:** I'm guilty of it too — scrolling through my phone late at night or binge-watching shows until my eyes start to water. But here's the truth: blue light is the enemy of good sleep! It messes with your melatonin levels and keeps you awake. So I make a

point of stepping away from screens at least an hour before bed. Instead, I pick up a book or do some light stretching.
- **Creating a Bedtime Routine:** I really can't stress this enough – having a calming routine sets the tone for sleep. Some nights, I just light a candle, play some soothing music, or even try a bit of meditation before bed. It's about telling your body, 'Hey, it's time to relax and unwind.' It could be as simple as reading a chapter of a book or jotting down a few thoughts in a journal.
- **Herbal Teas and Hot Beverages:** This one's become a little ritual for me. A warm cup of chamomile tea or even a cup of hot chocolate (yes, you heard that right) just before bed helps me feel relaxed and ready for sleep. I like to make it a part of my wind-down routine. Just like how a cosy blanket makes you feel at home, a soothing drink works wonders for your soul.

Sleep Is Not a Time Waster, It's an Investment

One thing I've learned over the years is that sleep is not a luxury – it's an investment. I used to feel guilty about needing a full eight hours. I'd think I was wasting time or missing out. But as I've grown older, I've come to embrace sleep as a non-negotiable part of my routine.

It regulates glucose levels, boosts immunity, helps long-term memory, detoxifies your body, and repairs it. The body releases different hormones during different stages of sleep, and when you don't get enough of it, it affects your entire endocrine system. Sleep is literally your body's way of getting to work behind the scenes, which is why it's essential for long-term health.

So yeah, a good night's sleep can improve your energy, brain function, and even your heart health. It reduces inflammation, helps your body store energy, and keeps you feeling happier and healthier. It's a long game, though – don't expect to make up for lost sleep just by napping for two days on the weekend. It doesn't work that way. Consistency is everything, and you need to prioritize sleep every night.

Sleep Tips

- **Create a Sleep-Friendly Environment:** Your bedroom should feel like a sanctuary. Keep it dark, cool, and quiet. You don't need a fancy sleep app to know that your body rests best when your surroundings are calm and comfortable.

- **Avoid the Late-Night Scroll:** I've completely cut social media out of my night-time routine. Scrolling through Instagram or getting into heavy conversations before bed only wires your brain. So now I steer clear of social media like the plague before bed.

The Power of the Nap

Let's talk about naps. Yes, they're underrated! If you can steal 15–20 minutes during the day to close your eyes, it's like hitting the reset button. Even when I'm on set or travelling, I've learned that those little moments of rest keep me balanced and energized. It's not about the length of time you nap; it's about allowing your body to rest and recharge for a burst of energy.

A power nap does wonders for your mental clarity and can help improve your productivity for the rest of the day. It recharges your mind and body, giving you the energy you need to continue with your tasks. I've found that these brief naps help me stay calm and focused, and more important, they boost my mood. Whether I'm in a trailer or taking a quick break at home, I try to get in those moments of quiet rest whenever I can. It's a game changer.

Magic Potion: Sleep, Water, Sunshine

Balance Your Workout, Diet, and Sleep for Maximum Results

I always say one hour of exercise is all you need. You don't have to live at the gym – just make that one hour count. Pair that with a good nutritious diet, and you're golden. But here's the catch: if you're eating right and training hard but skimping on sleep, it can undo all that effort. There's no point pushing yourself in the gym if you're staying up until 4 a.m. and undoing it all with poor sleep and food choices.

Sleep is the glue that holds your fitness and wellness efforts together. It's during deep sleep that your body repairs muscle tissue, rebuilds strength, and recovers from physical exertion. If you're not sleeping enough, your muscles don't get the chance to recover fully – and that slows down progress.

When you balance exercise, diet, and sleep, your body gets the time it needs to heal and grow stronger. The magic happens when you're consistent with these three essentials. Focusing on this trio instead of obsessing over unrealistic goals can have a far more profound impact on your overall well-being. And remember, overtraining doesn't mean better results. Prioritizing rest – especially quality sleep – ensures your body bounces back stronger every time.

How Sleep Affects Your Hair and Skin

Sleep and hormones are deeply connected, and this is where the real glow-up happens. When you're well rested, your cortisol (stress hormone) levels drop, reducing inflammation, oiliness, and hair loss. On the other hand, poor sleep sends those levels soaring, and the first place it shows is on your skin and scalp. That's when you get that dreaded combination of a dull complexion and limp, tired hair.

Sleep not only improves your skin's glow but contributes to hair health too. Deep sleep gives your body time to replenish hair follicles, restore skin cells, and regulate oil production. It helps maintain that glow, supports hair strength, and keeps breakouts and dullness at bay.

This becomes even more important during hormonal shifts – especially during periods, the perimenopause years, or times of heightened stress – when your body's natural rhythms need extra support. Poor sleep during these phases can lead to hair thinning, breakouts, and other signs of ageing. That's why getting quality, restorative sleep isn't just a beauty hack – it's a biological need. Deep sleep helps your body regulate hormones more effectively, bringing it back into balance from the inside out.

Yoga Asanas for Better Sleep

Yoga is one of my favourite ways to unwind and prepare for deep, restorative rest. It's not only great for flexibility and strength but also for calming the nervous system, releasing tension and clearing the mental clutter. Adding a few simple poses to your routine can make a world of difference in how well you sleep. These asanas work to stretch out tight areas, promote relaxation, and clear your mind after a busy day.

My Go-To Yoga Poses for Better Sleep

Supta Baddha Konasana
(Reclining Bound Angle Pose)
How to Do It
Sit on the floor with your legs extended. Bring the soles of your feet together, letting your knees fall open to the sides, and lie back. Place your arms on the floor, palms facing up. Close your eyes and breathe deeply for 5 to 10 minutes.

Benefits
This pose opens up the hips, calms the mind, and promotes relaxation – perfect for winding down.

Viparita Karani (Legs Up the Wall Pose)
How to Do It
Sit with one hip against a wall and slowly lie back, swinging your legs up the wall. Relax for 5 to 10 minutes, breathing deeply.

Benefits
Calms the nervous system, promotes circulation, and helps release stress.

Savasana (Corpse Pose)
How to Do It
Lie on your back with your legs extended and arms by your sides. Focus on deep breathing and let go of any tension for 5 to 10 minutes.

Benefits
A deeply restorative pose that helps release the stress of the day and prepares your body for sleep.

Ananda Balasana (Happy Baby Pose)
How to Do It
Lie on your back, pull your knees towards your chest, and hold your feet with your hands. Gently pull your knees down towards the floor and hold for 1 to 2 minutes.

Benefits
Stretches the back, relieves tension, and promotes relaxation before bed.

Pranayama (Breathwork for Relaxation)
How to Do It
Sit comfortably and inhale deeply through your nose, allowing your belly to rise. Exhale slowly through your mouth, extending the exhale. Breathe for 5 to 10 minutes.

Benefits
Activates the parasympathetic nervous system, calming your mind and preparing you for restful sleep.

Water: The Secret Elixir

Water. We've all heard it a million times, right? But honestly, I can't stress enough how essential it is. People talk about skincare routines, supplements, and treatments, but nothing – *absolutely nothing* – beats the power of water. It's my magic potion, the foundation of everything I do to stay healthy and glowing. Simple, yet so effective. No fancy serums or creams can replace the glow that comes from proper hydration.

And yes, I know I've already raved about hydration in the chapters on skin and hair. But hear me out: if there's one hill I'm willing to die on, it's this one. Even my editors couldn't convince me to stop talking about it. Why? Because it's *that* important.

For me, staying hydrated is the ultimate beauty hack. It's more than just drinking enough water – it's about supporting your body from the inside out. I've learned the hard way that dehydration really shows up in my skin and hair. I can feel it, and I can see it. So when I say water is my secret elixir, I *really* mean it!

Why Water Is Essential

First off, water is a detox champion. It flushes out toxins, keeps everything running smoothly, and helps your body stay in top shape. That means fewer breakouts and clearer skin, which is always a bonus. It also helps your immune system fight off infections, so you can say goodbye to those annoying colds that seem to sneak up on you. Plus, if you've ever had a headache after a long day, you'll know how much water can work its magic in soothing that.

But hydration doesn't stop at the physical. It plays a huge role in your sleep and mental well-being too. When you're well hydrated, your body doesn't have to work overtime, which means you're more likely to sleep better. And when your body gets the rest it needs, everything else falls into place. No more tossing and turning. Trust me, I've had my fair share of sleepless nights, and I know how much water plays a role in getting that quality, deep rest.

And here's the kicker: water can indeed improve your mood and cognition. When you're properly hydrated, you'll find that your brain functions better — you're sharper, more alert, and just overall in a better mood. If you're feeling sluggish or a little irritable, it's probably time to grab that water bottle. A few sips can seriously help lift your energy and keep you on top of your game. Just don't forget to keep sipping!

How Water Impacts Your Skin and Hair

Yes, I've touched on this before — but it's worth repeating because water *is* your skin and hair's best friend.

For Skin: Hydration is your best-kept beauty secret. When your skin is hydrated, it looks fresh, plump, and dewy. But when you're dehydrated? Oh boy. That's when the dryness and dullness start to creep in. Fine lines, rough texture — it all shows up when you're not drinking enough water. It's like your skin loses its glow, and no amount of expensive serums can bring it back if you're not taking care of your hydration. So, yes, water is your beauty filter!

For Hair: Just like skin, your hair thrives on hydration. I can always tell when I've skimped on water – my strands feel dry, frizzy, and lifeless (definitely not my vibe). Hydration helps maintain healthy growth, prevents breakage, and keeps your hair glossy. I've noticed that my hair is shinier and healthier when I'm properly hydrated. And when I fall short? Instant regret.

How Much Water Do You Really Need?

Everyone talks about the 2 to 3 litres a day rule, but here's the thing – I don't obsess over the exact amount. I listen to my body. Some days I need more, some days less. But the key is to drink consistently throughout the day. Carry a water bottle with you, and sip it regularly. I always make sure my bottle is within arm's reach, whether I'm at home, on set, or at a shoot. Hydration isn't about hitting a perfect number – it's about creating a habit. It's something you do for your future self. Not just for the glow, but for your mood, your focus, your sleep, and your energy.

Detox Recipes and Tips

So if you're now thinking, 'OK, hydration is cool – but I'm just not a fan of plain water,' let's make it fun. Before you reach for that can of cola or something processed or super sugary, here are a few easy ways to jazz it up:

- **Infused Waters:** Lemon, mint, cucumber, berries – it's like a spa day in a bottle. Hydration meets luxury. (You might remember this from the 'Skin' chapter, where I go deeper into my favourite glow shots and infusions.)
- **Detox Juices:** Green juices are my secret weapon – cucumber, spinach, lemon, ginger, mint. They hydrate, nourish, and detoxify all in one. These are my go-to when I need an energy boost or want to feel light and clean.
- **Water-Rich Foods:** Watermelon, strawberries, cucumbers, oranges – don't underestimate them. I snack on these throughout the day. It's the easiest, tastiest way to sneak in more hydration.

Think of this as your little hydration recap – just in case you needed the reminder. Because truly, hydration is non-negotiable. It's the simplest habit with the biggest impact. It supports every other choice you make for your health – your sleep, your skin, your workouts, your digestion, your energy.

Simple, easy, and oh-so-effective.

So here's my little tip: Drink up. Glow on. Thank me later!

Sunshine: Nature's Daily Dose of Wellness

Sunshine isn't just about getting that gorgeous golden glow – it's so much more. For me, it's like nature's ultimate reset button that energizes, uplifts, and nourishes my body from the inside out. It's one of my favourite daily rituals – it's free, easy, and has more benefits than you can imagine. Accessible and powerful, sunshine is a tool we often overlook, but one that has made a world of difference to my own well-being.

Sunshine and Bone Health: Why It Became Non-Negotiable

When I hit my forties, I started to feel a shift – not just in energy, but in how my body responded to everyday life. I was eating well, staying active, doing everything 'right', but still, I felt ... heavier. Not in weight, but in my bones. A certain stiffness, a fatigue that wasn't going away like it used to. That's when I began looking into what my body needed more of – and the answer was simpler than I expected: sunlight.

See, even the most calcium-rich diet needs a partner, and that partner is vitamin D. Our bodies naturally produce it when we're exposed to the sun, and it plays a critical role in helping us absorb calcium effectively. And you might have guessed why this decade of life brought me to that realization: like with everything else, our body's ability to absorb calcium decreases with age, and that's where sunlight comes in. So even if you're eating all the right things, it won't make much of a difference without enough vitamin D. That realization was a game changer for me.

A few years ago, I was on a long shoot – one of those hectic schedules where I was indoors all day, hopping from one location to another with barely a minute outside. After a few days, I noticed how off I felt: sluggish, sore, mentally foggy. I wasn't at my best, and I knew something was missing. That's when it hit me – I hadn't been out in the sun. No walks, no morning rays, not even 5 minutes of natural light.

Since then, I've made it a conscious habit to step outside every single day, even if it's just for a quick walk around the block or soaking in a few minutes of sunshine between takes. And the difference? It's incredible. I feel more grounded, more alive, and that heavy feeling in my body starts to melt away. It's not just about avoiding future bone issues – it's about feeling strong and supported in the present.

And here's a small ritual I love that makes the experience even better: I apply sesame oil to my skin before stepping out. It's rich in calcium and helps support vitamin D absorption while improving blood circulation. Plus, it keeps my skin nourished and protected – turning those few minutes in the sun into something far more intentional and restorative.

Sunshine, for me, isn't just a mood-booster. It's part of my daily wellness equation. Free, accessible, and far more powerful than we give it credit for – it's one of the simplest things I do to stay well, inside and out.

How Much Sun Do You Need?

Now timing is key when it comes to soaking in that sunshine. Ideally, aim for 10 to 15 minutes of sunlight exposure each day, but here's the important bit – avoid the afternoon sun, when the rays are at their harshest. The best time for sun exposure is either in the early morning or late afternoon, specifically before 9 a.m. or after 4.30 p.m. This is when the sun is gentler, and you can get all the benefits without the risk of overexposure or skin damage. I make it a point to step outside during these hours, even if it's just for a short walk. It's the best time to get the benefits without worrying about skin damage or the harsh UV rays that come in the middle of the day.

If you're busy and work indoors, a quick walk outdoors for 10 to 15 minutes during your lunch break can do wonders. It's amazing how a little sunlight, even in short bursts, can reset your mood, give you energy, and leave you feeling more balanced!

Sunshine and Menopause

For women, especially those navigating perimenopause and menopause, getting enough sunlight is even more critical. During these times, our hormones are all over the place, and let me tell you, that can throw us off balance. And here's what I've realized – sunshine helps. Vitamin D plays a major role in regulating hormones and preventing bone loss. It's like this natural ally that helps keep everything in check. So I always get my daily dose of sunlight, especially when I feel the shift in my energy or hormones. Sometimes all you need is a little sunlight to reset and balance things out.

Sun Protection Is Key

As much as I love soaking in some rays, I'm always careful about sun protection. You never want to overdo it, because sun damage can sneak up on you. Always apply sunscreen before heading out, especially if you're spending long periods in the sun. I also use UV-protectant hair products when I'm outdoors for long hours, especially on shoots. Your skin and hair need that extra layer of defence, so don't forget it!

The Essentials (Plus a Little Extra)

In a world full of shiny, new wellness routines, I always come back to the basics: sleep, water, and sunshine.

These three are my holy grail – the foundation of everything I do to stay grounded, balanced, and well. When I give them the attention they deserve, I can see the difference in how I feel, how I move, and how I show up every day. My energy is better, my skin glows, and my mood stays more even. No fancy product can replace that.

That said, there are times when life gets busy or my routine needs a little support. And that's when I turn to a few well-chosen supplements – not to replace the basics, but to gently enhance them.

Some of these, like collagen and omega-3, you've probably seen me talk about earlier – especially when it comes to skin and hair. I stand by them completely. Collagen, for instance, is part of my morning routine and works wonders for skin elasticity, hair strength, and even joint support. Omega-3s keep my skin hydrated and my heart happy – so they stay on my essentials list.

To that, I'd add two more staples:

Vitamin D: Especially during the colder months, when sunlight is limited, I take vitamin D supplements. It keeps my bones strong and supports my immunity – an absolute must.

Probiotics: Gut health is everything. A balanced gut not only improves digestion but also reflects in your skin, mood, and overall well-being. I take probiotics regularly to keep my system functioning smoothly.

Of course, none of these are magic pills – and they're not meant to replace the basics. They're more like my behind-the-scenes crew, supporting the lead cast of good sleep, hydration, and a little time in the sun. A little boost here and there, to keep things flowing and feeling good.

Keep it simple, stay consistent, and give your body what it truly needs. Everything else is just a bonus.

Final Word

In a world constantly chasing shortcuts and trending beauty fixes, I always return to the simplest, most powerful habits: sleep, water, and sunshine. They're not just part of my routine – they are the reason I feel centred, energized, and well. Prioritizing these three has changed the way I show up in my body and mind, and the glow that comes from that kind of alignment is unmatched. No miracle product can replace what these natural essentials give you. Start there, stay consistent, and you'll begin to notice the difference – subtle at first, and then all at once.

PART II

BODY

4
Food: Fuel for the Body and Mind

I've lost count of how many times I've been asked how I stay in shape, especially with all the food posts I share. Whether it's indulgent meals or foodie moments, there's an assumption that I must survive on air and some miracle diet. But if you've seen my reels or caught me behind the scenes on *Jhalak Dikhhla Jaa*, you know that's far from the truth. I'm a total foodie – it's in my blood! Yes, I have my cake, and I eat it too.

I don't overthink food. I don't stress about an extra hundred calories, nor do I eat an extra slice of pizza every day (though I enjoy it when I do!). The key is balance. I don't deny myself good food – after all, it's one of life's simple pleasures. I've learned to listen to my body and focus on moderation, without turning food into a source of stress. For me, it's about fuelling my body, supporting my energy, and feeling my best.

So what's my approach to food? How do I keep this balance? Let's break it down, starting with how I fuel my body, what's on my plate, and why it all works for me.

My Relationship with Food over the Years

Food has always been central to my family life. Growing up with a South Indian mother and a Punjabi father, I was surrounded by delicious food. From the comforting dosas and idlis my mom made to the hearty parathas and butter chicken my dad loved, I got the best of both worlds. Meals were never just about filling my stomach – they were about connecting with family, culture, and memories. That's still how I approach food today.

Living in Chembur, Mumbai, I was drawn to the vibrant world of Maharashtrian cuisine. Simple but incredibly flavourful meals like dal or sabzi/bhaji resonated with me deeply. My multicultural upbringing shaped not just what I eat but how I eat. Fresh ingredients, a love for spices, and the comfort of home-style cooking have become the soul of my kitchen. Food goes beyond nutrition for me. It's a reminder of my roots, and the love that goes into every meal.

Of course, it wasn't always this grounded. In my twenties, I could eat what I wanted without much thought. But as I got older, my perspective on food and my body began to shift. I realized that eating well wasn't just about chasing a goal weight. It was about energy, nourishment, and taking care of myself from the inside out. Like so many others, I got swept up early on in the media's obsession with extreme diets and 'quick fixes'. Paparazzi photos and their awkward angles made me self-conscious. A bit of cellulite, a bad shot, or a hint of bloating would send me into a spiral. I'd wonder, 'Is this what people think I look like?' I felt I wasn't living up to the 'perfect' image I thought I needed to project.

But over time, I realized that what I was criticizing in myself was just ... real. A little jiggle? Natural. Cellulite? Most women have it. Bloating after a meal? Normal. We aren't meant to look airbrushed or have washboard abs 24/7 – especially after a good meal! Honestly, a lot of it comes down to lighting, angles, and perspective.

The real shift came when I stopped trying to control my body. Health, I discovered, isn't about visible six-packs or impossible standards; it's about consistency, balance, and being kind to yourself. My relationship with food now centres on nourishment, not restriction. I enjoy the foods I love, honour my cravings, and trust my body to guide me. Over the years, I've embraced a holistic approach to eating, focusing on nourishing my body rather than chasing fleeting trends. A healthy relationship with food isn't about perfection; it's about tuning in, staying grounded, and choosing what supports me long-term.

Pregnancy and the Shift in My Food Approach

My twenties were a time of indulgence, and my metabolism could handle it. But pregnancy shifted my approach to food. The idea of 'eating for two' was often tempting, but I firmly believe in moderation. While I satisfied cravings when they came, I never let it go overboard. I focused on nourishing both my body and my baby with the right nutrients, avoiding overindulgence. Gaining unnecessary weight during pregnancy can cause long-term problems for both mother and child, and I wanted to ensure that wasn't the case. I made sure it was enough to stay healthy and strong while keeping my energy levels in check.

My Thirties: Nutrient-Dense Focus

In my thirties, the importance of nutrient-dense foods became clear to me. Gone were the days of relying on junk food and processed snacks. Instead, I focused on incorporating foods that would fuel me and keep my energy up. Lean proteins, whole grains, and plenty of vegetables became my go-to. I started thinking about food not just as a source of taste but as nourishment for my body, helping me to maintain energy for my career and personal life.

The Forties: Adjusting for My Changing Needs

As I moved into my forties, I noticed even more how food choices affected my body. With a slower metabolism and increased awareness of how food impacts my energy, I began adjusting my habits. One of the most notable changes was the introduction of intermittent fasting (IF). I've been practising it for years, but as I got older, I realized I needed to adjust my approach, especially considering hormonal shifts, to better align with my body's changing needs (more about this later). I continue to focus on nutrient-dense foods, prioritizing bone health, hormone balance, and immune support. I now make sure to include foods rich in vitamin D, omega-3s, and magnesium to support strength and overall wellness.

How I Balance My Diet

By now, you've probably gathered that balance is a big part of how I approach food – and life. After years of trial and error, I've learned that feeling good isn't about rigid rules or chasing perfection. It's about tuning in, trusting your body, and making choices that feel right for you. For me, that means no extreme restrictions or guilt trips around food. I don't cut out entire food groups, nor do I beat myself up for enjoying a rich meal. If I have something indulgent, like butter chicken or dessert, I simply balance it out the next day with a lighter meal or a little extra movement. It's this flexible, realistic rhythm that keeps me feeling my best – without turning food into something stressful.

Why Our Diet Needs to Evolve

When I think about the traditional diets our grandparents followed, I feel so much respect. They ate simple, whole foods with a strong focus on what was local and seasonal. Their meals were nourishing, and there was a connection to the earth. It was so intuitive. I still believe in those principles but also recognize that we live in a very different world now. What worked for our grandparents may not always work for us any more. The quality of food has changed drastically. Today, even grains, dairy, and fresh produce can carry preservatives or toxins, or be highly processed.

For instance, I used to consume dairy regularly, but now I'm much more mindful about its quality and consume it sparingly. Sugar too affects my skin and drains my energy. It's not just about how it affects my appearance – it's about how it makes me feel. And that's why balance and sustainability matter more than ever.

The Power of Simple, Balanced Plates

I've always gravitated towards meals that are simple, nourishing, and satisfying. Whole, fresh foods – seasonal vegetables, good-quality grains, and lean proteins – form the heart of my diet. I don't believe food needs to be complicated to be powerful. One of my all-time favourite meals? A rice bowl.

I remember this one particularly crazy day on set. I hadn't had time for a proper meal and threw together some rice, chicken, dal, and vegetables. That humble bowl, quick and wholesome, powered me through the rest of my shoot. At home, it's the same. I mix seasonal vegetables with rice, toss in a protein like tofu or grilled chicken, and that's dinner done. It's simple, it's real, and it works.

If reading that shocked anyone – good! It's high time we stopped demonizing simple carbs like rice. I've said it before and I'll say it again: rice has always been a staple in my life, and I don't feel guilty about it. Carbs give me the energy I need to function at my best. Skipping them leaves me feeling sluggish and off balance. For me, it's never about cutting them out;

it's about balancing them with vegetables, healthy fats, and protein. A bowl of rice with dal and sautéed greens? That's comfort, nourishment, and fuel – all in one.

And yes, protein is another non-negotiable for me. It helps me maintain muscle, keeps me full longer, and gives me sustained energy. I always make sure there's some in every meal – eggs, legumes, grilled meat, or even a handful of nuts. For hectic days, protein ladoos are a total lifesaver – quick to grab, not too heavy, and they give me the fuel I need without slowing me down.

This kind of eating isn't just about looking good, it's about feeling strong, grounded, and energized day in and day out.

Seasonal Eating: A Natural Approach to Balance

I believe in eating what's in season. Seasonal produce is often richer in nutrients and aligns better with our body's needs at different times of the year. In summer, I focus on hydrating fruits like melons, berries, and cucumbers, while in winter, I lean towards hearty vegetables like sweet potatoes and squash. These foods help me stay grounded and support my immune system. I also make sure to include leafy greens like palak (spinach) and methi (fenugreek) during the colder months, and fresh herbs like coriander and mint in the warmer months. Eating with the seasons just makes sense to me, and it's a practice that brings me closer to nature.

It's true that many fruits, especially those rich in natural sugars like mangoes and grapes, often get a bad rap and are labelled as 'too sugary' or 'unhealthy'. But I don't subscribe to that idea. Mangoes, for example, are loaded with vitamins, minerals, and antioxidants that benefit the body, and grapes have their own unique set of nutrients. I love incorporating these sweet fruits into my diet, but it's all about the timing and balance. I prefer eating them earlier in the day when my body can better process the natural sugars. To make them even more satisfying, I'll pair them with a little protein or healthy fats, like adding some nuts or a dollop of curd, which helps balance their glycaemic load. The trick lies in moderation, not in complete avoidance!

Hydration: The Foundation of My Health

You know by now that water is always at the base of my day, but I also believe in the detoxifying power of juices like karela, amla, and celery. Yes, karela juice might not be the easiest to drink, but it's helped me feel more energized and cleansed. Amla juice, on the other hand, is a staple for my skin and overall well-being. Alongside these juices, I drink ajwain and jeera water for their digestive benefits. I've learned that when my digestive system is in top shape, everything else – energy, skin, mood – falls into place.

Avoiding Raw Foods

I've learned to avoid raw food, especially when I'm eating out. Raw food, especially salads, doesn't always sit well with my digestive system, and I tend to fall sick more easily if I eat it. It's a personal choice, but it works best for me. When I'm dining out, I stick to cooked foods. There's no way of knowing where raw food has been handled or how well it's been washed, and I prefer to play it safe. A boiled sprout salad or a warm salad is my ideal choice when I'm out and about. It's all about being mindful of what my body needs, and for me, this approach ensures I stay healthy and feel good.

Striving for Consistency, Fixed Meal Times, and Portion Control

Maintaining consistency is crucial for me. I've found that eating at fixed times every day helps keep my energy levels steady and my metabolism in check. I try not to skip meals or eat too late, as I've learned that my body functions best with a routine. Sticking to meal timings has helped me avoid overeating or unnecessary cravings, and it keeps me in tune with my body's natural rhythm.

Another habit that's helped me stay consistent over time? I use the same-sized bowl for most of my meals. It naturally keeps my portions in check – no calorie counting, no overthinking. Just a simple visual cue that helps me stay balanced and satisfied.

Finding Balance, Day In and Day Out

You might be reading this and thinking, *'That's great for you, but how do I actually do this? I travel a lot, I don't have the time, and sometimes I don't know where to start.'*

Well, I get it! Talking about balance is one thing – living it every single day is something else entirely. But here's the thing: it's totally possible to stay on track and nourish your body, no matter what your schedule looks like. It just takes a bit of mindset work, a little prep, and a few simple, sustainable choices made consistently.

I'll be honest – it's not always easy. Some days I'm juggling shoots, travel, or back-to-back meetings; other days, I have the luxury of being at home. Each day looks different, and I adapt my meals accordingly. The goal is to find that sweet spot where I'm fuelling my body, staying energized, and making choices I feel good about, *without* getting caught up in the stress of doing it all 'perfectly'.

So, after all the advice and tips, here's a little peek into how it plays out in my day-to-day life. Do I really practise what I preach? (Well, I don't exactly 'preach', but you get the drift!)

A Regular Day: Simplicity and Consistency

On regular days, I keep my meals simple, nourishing, and easy to digest. I've found that whole foods – eggs, nuts and avocado, rice or millets, and lots of vegetables like carrots, beans, leafy greens, and mushrooms – help me stay energized without weighing me down. Hydration is always the first step: I start my day with a big glass of water, followed by my health shots and glow juices.

Breakfast sets the tone, so I rotate between my favourites – always leaning towards savoury meals that keep my energy stable through the day. I've found that starting with something protein-rich helps me avoid those mid-morning crashes. Most mornings, I'll go for a classic South Indian breakfast like idli or dosa, or have a paratha with ghee. Other days, I'll have avocado toast with eggs, or a moong dal chilla, or paneer bhurji with sautéed spinach. That said, I do have a sweet tooth! About once a week, I'll switch things up with a bowl of oatmeal topped with nuts, seeds, and seasonal fruit. It's a sweeter start, but still balanced — I focus more on the natural sweetness of fruit and avoid piling on unnecessary sweeteners. Sometimes, you just want a cosy bowl of oats, and that's totally OK.

Lunch is usually something wholesome but light — dal with rice and seasonal vegetables, rasam rice, or grilled chicken with greens. Often, I toss everything into a simple rice bowl with veggies and protein — it's my go-to comfort food that never fails. I've made peace with my love for rice; it's grounding and gives me sustained energy.

Dinner leans lighter. I might have grilled fish, a warm bowl of soup, or khichdi with sautéed veggies. If I'm craving comfort, I'll go for a small portion of dal makhani or butter chicken — these are occasional treats, not everyday staples.

Of course, not every day is perfectly structured. If I've had a heavier breakfast, I naturally balance it with a lighter lunch or dinner. If I'm hungrier than usual, I honour that — without guilt. It's not about strict rules or restrictions, but about making choices that support how I want to feel. That's the kind of balance I strive for: consistent, kind, and in tune with what my body needs.

Recommended Meal Plan for Regular Day

Time	Meal	Details
6.30 a.m.	Hydration	Glass of warm water with lemon or jeera water Detox shots (ginger, turmeric, lemon) Glow shots
7 a.m.	Pre-workout	Coconut water or plain water
8 a.m.	Post-workout	Protein shake with almond milk *or* Eggs with a handful of nuts or seeds
10.30 a.m.	Breakfast	Idli, dosa, or vegetable upma *or* Avocado toast with eggs *or* Oats porridge with nuts and berries *or* Moong dal chilla
1 p.m.	Lunch	Dal with rice and seasonal veggies *or* Grilled chicken with rice and spinach *or* Rice bowl with veggies and tofu or chicken

Time	Meal	Details
4 p.m.	Light Snack	Green tea with lemon *and* Fresh fruit (banana, apple, or kiwi) *and* Nuts (pistachios, walnuts, or pine nuts)
7 p.m.	Dinner	Grilled fish with vegetable stew *or* Khichdi with dal and sautéed veggies *or* Kati roll with grilled chicken or paneer
Before Bed	Hydration	Water with a splash of apple cider vinegar to aid digestion *or* Jeera water

A Day on Set or Travelling: Staying Prepared

When I'm travelling or working on a shoot, I adapt my routine to keep up with the pace, but the principle of balance stays the same. The first thing I do is pack my own snacks. I don't trust airline food, and I don't always know what's going to be available on set. I've had too many experiences where I'm faced with options that don't sit well with me or don't nourish my body in the way I need. I avoid relying on food that may be full of preservatives or additives. This has been essential for maintaining my health and energy levels, even when I'm on the move.

On a flight one day, I pulled out my homemade meal – a simple avocado and egg sandwich, some fruits, and infused water. The gentleman sitting next to me was shocked and asked, 'You eat that?' as if it was the worst thing in the world! I just laughed and said, 'Yes, I do.' Moments like that remind me how important it is to embrace what makes me feel good, even when it's not the 'trend' or the easiest option.

Meals during travel or shoots might look a little different depending on timing, but the focus remains the same: balance. Instead of opting for the heaviest, most calorie-laden items on a menu, I choose lighter options that nourish my body without overloading it. For breakfast or brunch, I often have an avocado and egg sandwich or a protein smoothie with banana and peanut butter. If I want something lighter, a moong dal chilla with paneer or eggs with a handful of nuts and seeds works well. For lunch, I'll grab a grilled chicken wrap or a quinoa salad with chickpeas, seasonal veggies, and tahini drizzle.

Even with the best planning, travel can be unpredictable. That's why I always carry snacks I know will fuel me – protein ladoos (made with oats, nuts, and dates), dried fruits, nuts, homemade chips, bananas, apples, or kiwis. These snacks are my lifesavers, especially in the late afternoons when I'm peckish or when I can't sit down for a full meal or can't find something healthy. They are energizing, help me avoid unhealthy options, and give me peace of mind, knowing I'm nourishing my body no matter where I am.

For dinner, I try to keep it simple and nourishing: prawn curry with rice or masala khichdi with buttermilk, or a quick bowl of grilled chicken with sautéed vegetables. It's about staying fuelled, no matter where I am.

Recommended Meal Plan for Busy Day (Shoot or Travel)

Time	Meal	Details
6.30 a.m.	Hydration	Glass of warm water with lemon or jeera water Detox shots (ginger, turmeric, lemon) Glow shots

Time	Meal	Details
10 a.m.–12 noon	Breakfast or Brunch	Avocado and egg sandwich with wholewheat bread *or* Protein-packed smoothie with banana, peanut butter, and flaxseeds
1–4 p.m.	Lunch	Grilled chicken or tofu wrap with veggies *or* Quinoa salad with chickpeas, seasonal veggies, and tahini drizzle
4 p.m.	Light Snack	Green tea with lemon *and* Fresh fruit (apple, banana, or kiwi) *and* Homemade protein ladoos or bars (oats, dates, nuts)
7 p.m.	Dinner	Prawn curry with rice *or* Masala khichdi with some chopped salad and buttermilk *or* Quick veggies with grilled chicken or paneer

Time	Meal	Details
Before Bed	Hydration	Water with a splash of apple cider vinegar to aid digestion *or* Jeera water

Rest Days: Flexibility and Enjoyment

Rest days are when I let things flow a little more naturally. There's less structure, fewer rules, and more room to simply *enjoy* food. I still eat wholesome meals, but I don't follow any fasting schedule or stick to a rigid plan. I wake up, tune in to how I'm feeling, and take it from there.

What's most important on rest days is giving myself permission to relax – not just physically, but mentally too. I still aim for balance, but I allow space for the occasional indulgence without guilt. If I'm craving something sweet or richer than usual, I'll have it, knowing I don't need to 'earn' it or 'burn it off' later.

So, like I said, food for me isn't about deprivation or extremes – it's about creating a rhythm that's nourishing, realistic, and rooted in self-awareness. Especially on rest days, that rhythm softens a little, making space for ease and enjoyment. Over time, I've learned that the best guide I have is my own body. Trends will come and go, but tuning in and responding with kindness? That's what truly lasts.

> ### For Women on the Go
>
> - **Prep Snacks:** Prepare protein ladoos, trail mix, or veggies to avoid junk food. They stay fresh for days and are perfect for busy moments.
> - **Mason Jars for Salads:** Layer salads in mason jars with dressing at the bottom. Shake it up when you're ready to eat!

Eat for Energy, Not for Trends

I'm sure that after hearing about my approach to eating, some of you may still be sceptical and may be thinking, 'OK, but what *is* her secret?' After all, most people assume that I follow some strict, elaborate diet to stay in shape — something expected of most celebrities. But here's the truth: I've tried my fair share of fad diets. I've chased the promises of quick fixes, like that early phase where I cut out all carbs, hoping to see fast results. Sure, I lost a bit of weight, but I also felt drained, sluggish, and irritable. My energy dipped, my mood suffered, and mentally I just wasn't in a good place. That's when it hit me: quick fixes come at a cost.

Whether it's extreme fasting, cutting out entire food groups, or eating next to nothing, these crash diets are simply unsustainable. You might see rapid weight loss for a few weeks, but at what cost? All you're left with is frustration, fatigue, and guilt. Over time, the weight comes back, and you're stuck in a cycle of restriction and self-inflicted punishment. That's no way to live!

I've realized that true health doesn't come from chasing the latest trend. Over time, I've experimented with different eating styles, like trying veganism or not eating onion, tomato, and garlic. Did I notice any significant changes? Not really! Everyone's looking for that 'secret' formula for weight loss, but here's the truth: there's no magic formula. True wellness is about finding what works *for you* and building a sustainable, healthy relationship with food. For me, it's no longer about following the newest fad. It's about nourishing my body with balanced meals that keep me energized, healthy, and feeling my best.

So what actually works? Three simple principles: moderation, listening to your body, and eating smaller, more frequent meals. These have helped me build a healthy, balanced lifestyle. Here's how:

- **Moderation over Deprivation.** Carbs, fats, proteins – they're all essential. I don't believe in vilifying food groups. I eat carbs for fuel, fats for healthy cells, and protein for strength. It's not about avoiding them; it's about portion, timing,

and pairing them smartly. Balance isn't boring – it's liberating. When you know you *can* eat everything, you stop obsessing over food.
- Listen to Your Body. Over the years, I've learned to trust my body. I don't count calories or weigh every bite – I tune in to how I'm feeling. Had a heavy breakfast? Then I'll go for a lighter lunch. Extra hungry one day? I eat a little more. It's that simple.
- Food Shouldn't Be a Punishment. It should feel good. Like that day on set when I was happily eating a bowl of rice and dal and someone asked, 'You eat that?' I smiled and said, 'Of course.' You don't need anyone's approval for your food choices – just your own comfort and confidence.
- Have Small, Frequent Meals. I used to fall into the trap of skipping meals and then bingeing later. It never felt good. What works for me now is eating smaller meals regularly throughout the day. It keeps my metabolism steady, prevents energy crashes, and supports better digestion. Consistent nourishment beats extremes every single time.

The bottom line? Trust your body. Nourish it consistently and avoid the traps of restrictive diets. There's no shortcut, no cleanse, no restriction that's worth sacrificing your peace of mind or your long-term health. For me, building a lasting relationship with food is about listening to my body and focusing on long-term wellness. The real secret? *Balance.* It's not glamorous, but it works – and it lasts.

Cutting Through the Noise

- Social media nutrition advice can be misleading – don't get swept up by every trend.
- Focus on reliable, credible sources like registered dietitians or nutritionists who promote balanced, sustainable approaches.
- Follow experts you trust – Rujuta Diwekar's advice is a great example of a sensible approach to nutrition.
- Don't jump on every new diet trend. Give it time to show real results.
- If a diet feels too extreme or doesn't suit you, it probably isn't the right fit. Listen to your body.
- Tailor your approach to your lifestyle – make simple, sustainable changes that work for *you*.
- Remember: anything unsustainable will eventually fail. Keep it real, trust the process, and listen to your body.

What I Eat for Radiant Skin and Hair

By now we've established that beauty starts from within. But what exactly does that mean when it comes to food? Over the years, I've learned that a nutrient-packed, well-balanced diet isn't just about getting a great body; it's the key to fabulous skin and shiny hair. And the best part? You don't need miracle ingredients or the latest trendy superfood. Simple, wholesome meals can work wonders when chosen with intention.

So here's a list of the foods I return to again and again – some I've already talked about and some new. These are my absolute go-tos for glowing skin and healthy hair. Think of this as your glow-up grocery list – nothing fancy, just the good stuff your body and beauty will love.

- **Berries:** Antioxidants galore! These beauties fight oxidative stress and keep my skin glowing. In smoothies, as snacks, or just on their own – they're a must.
- **Avocados:** Healthy fats for hydration. My skin and hair love them. I pop them on toast, throw them into salads, or just scoop them straight up.
- **Leafy Greens:** Spinach, kale, methi – these are packed with vitamins and minerals that do wonders for both skin and hair. Whether in a smoothie or a curry, they're always in my diet.

- **Nuts and Seeds:** My energy-boosting snack of choice. Rich in protein and healthy fats, these powerhouses keep me full and satisfied without the sugar crash.
- **Turmeric:** My go-to anti-inflammatory. It's the magic ingredient in my chai, smoothies, or curries – helping me maintain that healthy glow from within.
- **Omega-3-Rich Foods:** Flaxseeds, chia seeds, and the occasional fatty fish keep my skin hydrated and my hair strong. Hydration is key, and omega-3 works wonders.
- **Fruits:** I'm all about fruits rich in vitamin C – think oranges, papayas, and kiwis. These are collagen boosters that keep my skin firm and glowing.
- **Amla (Indian Gooseberry):** Amla juice is my little secret. It's packed with vitamin C and antioxidants – hello, glowing skin!
- **Celery Juice:** Great for detoxifying, and it's a must for healthy, clear skin. It helps flush out toxins and keeps things in balance.
- **Karela (Bitter Gourd):** Not everyone's favourite, but karela juice is a game changer. Detoxifies and helps clear the skin. It's a little bitter but totally worth it with a dash of honey!

For me, eating these nutrient-dense foods has made a massive difference. But let's be real. It's not just about adding the good stuff in, it's also about cutting out what doesn't serve me. Sugar? A big no-no. It causes inflammation, which leads to breakouts and dull skin. I keep it in check because, honestly, who needs that.

So the secret to glowing skin and healthy hair? Simple. Feed your body the right fuel, and it will work its magic. If you want to glow, start by giving your body the nutrients it craves, and the results will be impossible to miss.

Snack Smarter: Hacks to Avoid Bingeing

Snacking can be a double-edged sword – especially after a long day or when stress kicks in. I totally get it! But here's the thing: **snacking isn't bad** – even if you're following a nutritionist-recommended plan. In fact, it's a smart way to keep your energy steady and avoid reaching the point where you're starving and end up bingeing. The key is to do it mindfully, with a little planning and balance.

Here's how I snack smarter and avoid the pitfalls:
- **Mindful Meals:** I start by ensuring my dinner has a solid balance of protein, healthy fats, and complex carbs. This keeps me full and satisfied,

reducing cravings. Example: Grilled chicken, veggies, and quinoa or sweet potato.
- **Healthy Snacks Between Meals:** When hunger strikes before dinner, I reach for nourishing snacks like:
  - A handful of almonds or roasted chickpeas.
  - Green tea with a squeeze of lemon.
  - A banana or apple for a quick energy boost.
- **Stay away from Sugary Snacks:** A few years ago, during a late shoot, I swapped sugary snacks for a small bowl of poha with nuts. It was so satisfying, and I didn't feel bloated or sluggish after – definitely a game changer!
- **Avoid Late-Night Eating:** Eating too late can disrupt sleep. My personal rule: No eating after 7 p.m., allowing my body time to digest and rest. On weekends, I'll indulge, but during the week, I stick to this routine. If I've had a heavy lunch, I'll opt for a lighter dinner (grilled fish and soup or a vegetable stew).
- **Sweet-Tooth Fix:** I satisfy my cravings without the sugar crash by opting for:
  - Dried fruit or curd with a handful of mixed berries (frozen or fresh) and chia seeds.
  - A small piece of dark chocolate.

- A homemade protein bar made with oats, dates, and nuts.
- **Carry Healthy Snacks:** I always pack options like roasted chickpeas, almonds, or homemade granola. This way, I avoid unhealthy temptations when I'm out and about.
- **Eat Before Going Out:** When I'm heading to a party or social gathering, I eat something light beforehand to line my stomach – like eggs, idlis, or avocado toast. This way, I'm not starving when I arrive and can avoid overindulging.
- **Apple Cider Vinegar (ACV):** I take a shot of diluted ACV, either before a heavy meal or after indulging. It helps balance blood sugar, aids digestion, and reduces bloating.

With these hacks, I can indulge without going overboard and keep my energy levels steady through the day. It's not about restricting – it's about being mindful and prepared.

Intermittent Fasting: A Mindful Approach to Eating and Recharging

If you're wondering whether there's a secret behind how I manage to stay energized, focused, and light on my feet, it's not really a secret. It's a simple, science-backed rhythm that I've found works wonders for my body: intermittent fasting.

It's not about jumping on a trend or following something blindly. For me, IF is about giving my body the time it needs to reset. When we fast for extended hours, typically anywhere between 14 and 18 hours, our body gets a break from constant digestion and switches gears. During this time, it starts tapping into stored fat, regulating blood sugar, reducing inflammation, and even triggering a cellular clean-up process known as autophagy. It's something I learned through my own practice and from nutritionists I trust, and I've felt the benefits first-hand.

Here's how I've made it work for me:
- **My Personal Routine:** I follow an 18:6 fasting window. I usually eat dinner by 7 p.m. and break my fast around 1 p.m. the next day. This gives my body time to rest and reset, and I genuinely feel lighter and more in tune with myself.
- **Morning Workouts on an Empty Stomach:** I prefer working out before I eat. It might sound intense, but I've noticed better focus and clarity when I train fasted. It helps set the tone for my day.
- **First Meal:** When I break my fast, I go for a hearty, nutrient-packed meal. I make sure it

includes protein, healthy fats, and fibre to keep me full and energized through the afternoon.
- **Flexibility Is Key:** Over the years, I've adjusted my routine based on what my body needs. These days, I fast every other day. And during my menstrual cycle, I don't fast at all. It's important to stay aware and not push yourself unnecessarily. Listening to your body matters more than sticking to a schedule.

Finding Your Own Routine: It's All About Listening to Your Body

Intermittent fasting isn't a one-size-fits-all formula. It's about experimenting and discovering what rhythm works best for you. If you're just starting out, don't be afraid to play around with different windows.
- Some people thrive on a 16:8 window (16 hours of fasting, 8 hours of eating), while others prefer a gentler 14:10 approach. I do 18:6, but that's not a rule – it's just what works for me.
- No matter the window, it's important to break your fast with intention. Choose whole, nutrient-rich foods – think protein, fibre, and healthy fats – to give your body the fuel it deserves after the fast.
- IF isn't just about weight management. It's about overall well-being. I've found that I feel

more energized, less bloated, and more mentally focused when I'm in my groove with fasting. It also helps regulate blood sugar and supports digestion, which makes a big difference in how I feel throughout the day.

Should You Try Intermittent Fasting?

That's entirely up to you – and your body. IF has worked beautifully for me, but it's not meant for everyone.

If you have thyroid issues, PCOD, diabetes, or if you're pregnant, breastfeeding, or prone to disordered eating, I'd strongly recommend checking with a doctor or nutritionist before starting. Hormones, blood sugar levels, and overall energy can be sensitive to long fasting windows – especially for women. What feels great for someone else might not suit your body, and that's OK.

As I say, if something feels off, it probably is. Fasting should feel energizing – not depleting. If you're constantly tired, moody, or dizzy, take a step back and reassess. Nothing is worth compromising your health.

Not About Deprivation, but About Timing

What I love most about IF is that it's not about eating less – it's about **eating smarter**. It helps me tune into my natural hunger cues and avoid mindless snacking.

More than anything, it's helped me build a better relationship with food. I'm not eating just because the clock says so or out of boredom – I eat because I want to nourish myself.

So if IF feels right for you, give it a try. If not, that's OK too. It's not a badge of honour – it's just one of many tools that can help us live a little more mindfully. As always, the goal isn't perfection – it's awareness, balance, and feeling good in your own skin.

From Chembur to Scarlett House

I've always believed that good health and energy come from nourishment, not deprivation. As my metabolism has changed with age, I've learned to focus on meals that nourish my body, keep me energized, and help me stay mindful. This approach has not only shaped my personal eating habits but also the menu at my restaurant, Scarlett House.

At Scarlett House, we focus on wholesome, satisfying meals that are easy on the system and nourishing. The dishes are a reflection of everything I value about food – balance, simplicity, and nourishment. Here's a taste of some of my favourite items on the menu:

- **Malabar Prawn Curry:** A spicy, aromatic dish that takes you straight to the coast.

- **Banana Peri Peri Fries:** A fiery twist on a classic snack.
- **Podi Chutney Sushi:** South Indian flavours meet sushi – a light, fresh fusion.
- **Madras Beet Maki Rolls:** Fresh and full of taste, bursting with nutrition.
- **Fig and Burrata Salad:** The perfect mix of creamy, tangy, and sweet.
- **Thecha Paneer:** A nod to my Maharashtrian roots (recipe below).
- **Masala Khichdi:** Comfort food made simple and nourishing.

These dishes embody my food philosophy – foods that make you feel good from the inside out. And the beauty of it? They're easy to recreate at home. Here are some recipes inspired by my food journey.

Thecha Paneer

This dish is a comforting and flavourful reminder of my Maharashtrian heritage, and I try to have it whenever I can. It's simple, flavourful, and brings me right back to my roots in Chembur. Here's how I make it:

Ingredients
- 200 g paneer (cottage cheese), cut into cubes
- 4–5 green chilies
- 4–5 garlic cloves
- 2 tbsp roasted peanuts
- A handful of fresh coriander leaves and stems
- Salt to taste
- 1 tbsp oil

Method
- Begin by dry-roasting the green chilies, garlic cloves, and peanuts in a pan over medium heat until they become aromatic. Keep stirring to ensure they don't burn.
- Once roasted, coarsely grind together the chilies, garlic, peanuts, and fresh coriander leaves and stems using a mortar and pestle or a grinder. Add salt to taste.
- Heat oil in a pan and sauté the paneer cubes until they turn golden brown on all sides.
- Add the prepared thecha to the pan with the paneer and toss everything together so the paneer is well-coated with the flavourful paste.
- Garnish with fresh coriander leaves. Serve hot with roti or rice.

Protein-Packed Breakfast Smoothie

Ingredients
- 1 scoop of protein powder (plant-based or whey)
- ½ banana
- 1 tbsp peanut butter
- 1 tbsp flaxseeds
- 1 cup almond milk (or any plant-based milk)
- A dash of cinnamon and turmeric

Method
- Add all the ingredients – protein powder, banana, peanut butter, flaxseeds, almond milk, cinnamon, and turmeric – into a blender.
- Blend until smooth and creamy. Adjust the consistency by adding more milk if needed.
- Pour into a glass and enjoy this nutrient-packed breakfast to kick-start your day with energy and protein.

My Favourite Rice Bowl

Ingredients
- 1 cup cooked rice (brown rice or white rice)
- ½ cup grilled veggies (carrot, zucchini, bell peppers)

- 1 boiled egg or grilled chicken
- A handful of spinach
- 1 tbsp olive oil for dressing
- Salt, pepper, and lemon juice to taste

Method

- Begin by cooking your rice. You can use either brown or white rice, depending on your preference.
- Grill or sauté your vegetables until they are tender and slightly charred.
- Boil an egg or grill some chicken to your liking. If you prefer plant-based, tofu works great too.
- In a bowl, layer the rice, veggies, and protein. Add a handful of fresh spinach to the bowl.
- Drizzle olive oil over the bowl, and season with salt, pepper, and a squeeze of lemon juice to taste.
- Mix everything together and enjoy a balanced, satisfying meal that provides protein, fibre, and healthy fats.

Easy and Healthy Kati Roll

Ingredients
- 1 wholewheat wrap
- 1 serving of grilled chicken or paneer
- Lettuce or any leafy greens
- Slices of cucumber, tomato, and onion
- Tahini dressing or hummus
- Salt and black pepper to taste

Method
- Start by warming the wholewheat wrap in a skillet or microwave until it's soft and pliable.
- Grill your choice of protein (chicken or paneer) and slice it into bite-sized pieces.
- Lay the wrap flat and add a layer of leafy greens, such as lettuce or spinach, followed by the grilled chicken or paneer.
- Top the protein with fresh slices of cucumber, tomato, and onion for crunch and flavour.
- Drizzle tahini dressing or hummus on top, and season with salt and black pepper to taste.
- Roll it up tightly. Serve with a side of lemon wedges for a fresh, tangy kick.

Final Word

You've probably heard me say this before — but balance and moderation truly are the cornerstones of how I eat and live. Food isn't about deprivation or chasing quick fixes. It's about finding a sustainable rhythm that nourishes your body, supports your goals, and fuels you through whatever life brings.

Over the years, I've come to trust one thing above all: my body. I've never been one for fad diets or drastic cleanses. Instead, I've found that long-term health comes from consistency, simplicity, and tuning in — building habits that support how I feel, day in and day out.

Food is more than just fuel — it's a form of self-care. When you nourish your body with real, whole foods and treat it with kindness, it gives back in energy, vitality, and glow. So keep it simple, make mindful choices, and enjoy every bite. Because in the end, food should be a celebration — of life, of health, and of yourself.

5

Fitness: More Than Just a Look

I've been in the industry for decades, and believe me, it's far from a nine-to-five job. Long hours, constant travel, demanding shoots, events ... it's physically intense, and no two days are ever the same. Staying fit isn't a luxury for me, it's a necessity. If I didn't make fitness a part of my daily routine, I simply wouldn't be able to keep up with the pace, stay sharp, and show up fully.

When I started out, my fitness goals were very different. I was focused on appearances – losing weight for a shoot, chasing a certain physique, stressing over how I looked in a bikini. Managing the number on the scale or fitting into a dress size were my biggest stressors. It's easy to get caught up in aesthetics, especially in this industry. But over time, something shifted.

Gradually, I began to see fitness as something much bigger and more enduring. It became the foundation of everything I do. It keeps me energized, grounded, and mentally strong. I stopped seeing it as just a tool for transformation and started embracing it as a way of life. Of course, it still makes me feel good about my body. But today, I no longer wake up to work out just to stay 'in shape'. I move because it fuels my day and helps me feel strong, capable, and alive.

It's not about bouncing back or achieving perfection. It's about building strength that lasts, so I can keep up with my demanding line of work, stay present for my family, and show up for myself. I've learned that it's not about doing it all; it's about doing it consistently. It's an ongoing journey, and I'm committed to it, day in and day out. Whether it's a shoot, a yoga class, or a long-haul flight across time zones, staying active gives me the stamina to be my best self and find balance, no matter how hectic life gets.

The Evolution of My Fitness Journey: From Early Years to Today

Laying the Foundation: Childhood and Teenage Fitness

Looking back at my childhood, I realize how those early years were the foundation of my fitness journey. It wasn't about structured gym workouts or rigorous training plans; it was simply about staying active and having fun. My family encouraged an outdoor lifestyle. I wasn't the type to stay indoors glued to the TV. I loved being outside, playing sports, running around, or riding my bike around the neighbourhood.

There was a sense of freedom in those days – no fitness goals, no timelines, just the joy of movement.

One thing that sticks out is my deep love for running. As a teenager, I got involved in track and field, and I competed in local events. It was exhilarating to feel the wind in my hair as I ran. But alongside this, I found myself drawn to dancing. It began with Bharatanatyam, ballet, and jazz ballet. For me, dance was not only an art form but also a serious physical activity that kept me fit. I used to dance in a studio with other kids, and we'd sweat it out for hours, working through routines.

The few years I spent training taught me discipline, control, and balance. It gave me a deep understanding of how the body moves, the importance of posture and agility, and how flexibility and strength must work hand in hand. That foundation stayed with me as I moved into adulthood and helped me realize that fitness isn't just about building strength – it's about nurturing the body's natural balance.

Fitness in My Twenties: The Shift to Goal-Driven Workouts

Aerobics was a big craze in the early 1990s and I got hooked on it because it reminded me so much of dance – it was all about working out to music, having fun, and just sweating it out. Of course, now we have Zumba, but back then, aerobics was the craze. We'd put on music, let loose, and work up a sweat for an hour or so, and it was amazing. It was the same kind of release I'd get from dancing, just in a more structured workout format.

In my twenties, fitness became a professional necessity. Working in the entertainment industry, I quickly realized that staying in top shape wasn't just a personal choice but a part of the job. The demands of shoots, performances, and long hours meant I had to stay lean, energetic, and strong to keep up.

One of my first major shoots was for my debut music video for 'Gud Naal Ishq Mitha'. The choreography was simple but the retakes demanded stamina. But it was 'Chaiyya Chaiyya' that truly pushed my limits. Dancing on top of a moving train under the blazing sun was an unforgettable challenge. To prepare, I focused on dance-based cardio and building cardiovascular endurance. More than appearances, it was about having the strength to perform at my best, even under such extreme conditions. 'Maahi Ve' for *Kaante* was another test, for not only did I have to attempt pole dancing, I had to make it look effortless while engaging my core.

Each music video presented its own set of challenges, but the focus was always the same: staying fit and ready for whatever the shoot demanded. I remember constantly experimenting with dance-based workouts to stay at my best. At the time, my fitness was goal-oriented: looking my best for a role, staying lean for a shoot, or meeting the demands of a performance.

Rebuilding After Pregnancy: The 'Kaal Dhamaal' Shoot

I didn't actually step into a gym with the intent to lose weight until after I gave birth, at the ripe age of 27. Giving birth to my son, Arhaan, was one of the most transformative periods of my life. I had always been active – dance, daily movement, you name it. I was flexible, agile, and strong. Dance had already provided me with rigorous training, from warm-ups to performance-ready conditioning. But after pregnancy, I knew I needed to take a new approach to get my body back into shape.

That said, the changes I went through were a real eye-opener – physically and emotionally. In the first few months of pregnancy, I remember looking in the mirror and feeling so disconnected from my body. It wasn't easy seeing how different I looked, and at first, it was hard to reconcile with this new version of myself. But I wasn't in a rush. I told myself that it would take time, and I had to be patient.

During pregnancy, I stayed active, but I knew I had to be mindful. I wasn't doing anything extreme:

I walked every single day for an hour without fail. Sometimes I'd drag a friend or family member along to keep me company. My walks were my time to unwind and catch up with loved ones. And don't get me wrong, I was strict about going to my Lamaze classes and staying engaged in my fitness. I didn't want to overdo it, but I wanted to make sure my body remained active and strong. The idea of being sedentary just wasn't in me.

Then, after Arhaan was born, I had to figure out the best way to transition back into fitness. It wasn't going to happen overnight, and I knew that. I also had to go back to my job at MTV. I slowly started adding gentle stretches, short walks, and reintroducing yoga into my routine. But it wasn't just about losing the baby weight. I wanted to regain my strength and feel good about myself. About eight months post-delivery, I had a shoot for 'Kaal Dhamaal' in the film *Kaal*. It was a huge challenge, as I wasn't the same person I was before pregnancy. I couldn't just jump into extreme workouts, especially with my body still adjusting to the changes. But I didn't back down. I kept moving forward, starting with weight training and cardio, even though I was breastfeeding. I felt so committed to regaining my strength that breastfeeding didn't stop me. In fact, it made me feel connected to my body in a way I wasn't before. I started to take things slowly and listen to what my body needed.

I had to get my body ready for a music video, and seeing stretch marks or dealing with my body's changes wasn't easy. But I learned a lot about patience. There were days when I couldn't do things I once could, and my body resisted in ways it never had before. But I didn't rush. I accepted that I couldn't push too hard, too fast. Somewhere along the way, I started appreciating what my body had gone through and what it was still capable of. I remember walking onto that set, feeling so proud of how far I had come. Sure, my body had changed, but it had become stronger and more resilient.

If you've recently had a baby, remember there's no rush to get back to your old body. Start slow, listen to your body's pace, and focus on recovery. The journey is different for everyone, and that's OK.

The Thirties: Discovering Yoga and the Power of Slowing Down

In my thirties, I needed a shift. That's when fitness became a tool to manage stress and stay grounded in a hectic career, where the dynamic pace, constant travel, and back-to-back shoots were starting to take a toll on my body. This shift was only made clearer when I suffered a dance injury. It wasn't major, but it forced me to reassess my approach to fitness. I realized I couldn't keep pushing my body without listening to it.

I could no longer hit the gym regularly. That's when yoga came in. Yoga wasn't something I had embraced in my younger years. I always thought it was too slow for me. But as my body started feeling tighter and more strained, I realized yoga was exactly what I needed.

The first time I seriously practised yoga, I could feel a shift in how I approached my body and movement. It wasn't about pushing harder or lifting more – it was about tuning in to my body's needs, slowing down, and focusing on the breath. Yoga became the anchor that helped me reconnect with my body and regain a sense of peace. It gave me flexibility, mental clarity, and the space to breathe and reset, and taught me mindfulness.

Yoga complemented my cardio and weight training routine and eventually became a daily practice, something I relied on not only for its physical benefits but also for the emotional peace it brought me.

The Forties: Embracing New Realities

Turning 40, I realized that my body was no longer the same as it was in my twenties and thirties. Things didn't feel as firm; it was easier to put on weight and harder to shed. But instead of feeling discouraged, I used this as fuel to push myself in a different way. The changes in my body weren't a setback – they were an opportunity to embrace a more sustainable approach to fitness.

I've learned to listen even more closely to my body and approach my fitness routine with more patience and wisdom. I no longer try to push through pain or exhaustion. I respect my limits. Recovery, stretching, and foam rolling became just as important as strength training and yoga. I had to stop expecting my body to perform the way it did when I was younger. I no longer aim for the same physical appearance; instead, my focus is on functional strength, longevity, flexibility, and building stamina and strength that will serve me for years to come.

But turning 40 also made me more driven than ever. I knew that after this age, things would change – everything starts to feel like gravity is working against it, and your body reminds you that it's not as forgiving. So I pushed myself even harder. I didn't just accept these changes; I embraced them, and made fitness and wellness my new goal. I pushed myself like never before, even though I knew that losing those last few kilos would be harder. The hormones, the internal changes – everything seemed to work against me, but I wasn't ready to give in. Instead, I became more unstoppable.

The goal now isn't to look the way I did in my twenties; it's to be strong, capable, and healthy. I want to challenge myself, but in a way that's sustainable and that honours my body's needs.

Looking Ahead to 50

As I move closer to 50, I know that my fitness routine will continue to evolve. With age comes a greater focus on bone health and joint care, particularly to counter the risks of osteoporosis and other age-related challenges. Flexibility and balance, which have always been important to me, are now even more crucial as they help maintain mobility and prevent injuries. Perimenopause has also brought new considerations into my fitness routine – weight management can be trickier, and it's important to listen to my body's changing needs. While I know that challenges lie ahead, I'm prepared to face them with the same mindfulness and consistency that have kept me going for all these years. My goal now is longevity – not just to look good but to remain strong, flexible, and healthy so that I can continue doing what I love well into the future.

Morning Rituals: Setting the Tone for the Day

As a morning person, I've learned that starting my day with some form of movement is non-negotiable. It sets the tone for everything that comes after. My mornings are sacred — it's when I am my most energized, and it's when I dedicate time to my fitness routine. Whether it's a strength training session, yoga, or a quick cardio workout, I always start with movement. The variety in my routine keeps it exciting and fresh, and it's important for me to switch things up based on what my body needs on any given day. I don't like to stick to a rigid workout schedule. Instead, I focus on balancing different types of exercises, keeping my body engaged and guessing.

On some days, I'll dive into yoga — focusing on flexibility, breathing, and mindfulness. Other days, I'll prioritize strength training to build muscle or focus on Pilates to maintain core strength and flexibility. And yes, there are days when a simple walk, a swim, or a good stretch does wonders. It's about listening to my body and tuning in to what feels right. I don't believe in forcing a workout when it doesn't feel right, but I always make sure I show up. Even if it's just a short session, I make it a point to move.

My morning routine also includes hydration, vitamin shots, and some light wellness rituals, which keep me grounded and ready to take on the day. These little rituals, although simple, help prepare my body and mind for what's ahead.

Adaptability: Fitness on the Move

When my schedule is packed with shoots or travel, maintaining a workout routine can be challenging. But I've learned how to adapt. I keep workout gear in my bag always. On shoot days or during travel, when a full workout isn't feasible, I sneak in a few stretches, take a walk around the block, do a quick set of squats between takes, or practise a short yoga sequence in my hotel room. Staying active is about being adaptable. When time is limited, I find moments to fit in movement, and that consistency helps me stay on track, no matter where I am or what I'm doing.

The key takeaway is that it's not about finding time – it's about making time for movement, no matter what the circumstances are.

Mind, Body, Strength: A Holistic Approach to Fitness

My fitness routine isn't just about one thing. It's a blend of yoga, Pilates, and weight training – each serving a unique purpose and complementing the other. Yoga gives me flexibility, calm, and a deep sense of control, while Pilates focuses on building that core strength that's essential for everything I do. Weight training, on the other hand, is all about building muscle and strength that supports both the yoga and Pilates practices. The integration of all three keeps me fit and strong, ensuring that I'm not focusing on only one aspect of fitness but nurturing my body in all respects. It's about being strong, flexible, and resilient, no matter what life throws my way.

Role of Yoga in My Fitness Regimen

Yoga has been the cornerstone of my fitness routine. It's not just an exercise to me; it's a practice that has transformed me both physically and mentally. I discovered yoga when I was recovering from a significant injury, and it became the key to my recovery. Before yoga, I was used to pushing my body through high-intensity workouts, lifting heavy weights, and relentlessly working to achieve physical goals. But yoga taught me a new way to move, to listen to my body, and to honour it, rather than just pushing through the pain.

When I started practising yoga, I struggled with flexibility and couldn't even touch my toes. I was sceptical at my first yoga class. I thought, 'How can slow stretches and deep breathing help me?' But as I began to feel the shift in my body, I realized how yoga was healing me, not just physically, but emotionally. From there, I made yoga a part of my daily routine. The deeper benefits of yoga – mental clarity, mindfulness, and connection to my body – became apparent almost immediately. Today, I can do full backbends, inversions, and flows, which once seemed impossible.

Yoga has completely reshaped my body, my mind, and my spirit. It has helped me recover from injuries, improve my strength, and maintain flexibility. But most important perhaps, it's my tool during stressful times, helping me stay calm, centred, and balanced. Yoga provides me with a sense of calm and mental clarity that no other form of exercise has been able to replicate.

Why Yoga Is More Than Just Exercise

For me, yoga is a blend of everything I love about fitness. I get to combine weights, stretches, asanas, and even elements of Pilates – all in one practice. Yoga gives me that grounding I crave, and the best part is, I get to do it barefoot. The connection to the ground, the earth beneath me, is deeply therapeutic. It's almost like grounding myself with Mother Nature. When I first started, I was sceptical about meditation. But I've realized that yoga is itself a form of meditation. The deep breathing, the focus on each movement – it's all meditative.

We often underestimate the power of breathing. But every deep breath, every mindful inhale and exhale, is invigorating. It fills me with energy and helps me refocus. In fact, breathing exercises have become a crucial part of my routine. I start every yoga session with pranayama – it's my way of connecting my mind and body, clearing my thoughts, and finding mental balance.

There are five main breathing techniques I incorporate into my routine, and each one serves a unique purpose.

1. Bhastrika (Bellows Breath): This invigorating breathing technique increases oxygen flow, energizes the body, and clears the mind.
2. Anulom Vilom (Alternate Nostril Breathing): A calming practice that balances the left and right hemispheres of the brain, reduces stress, and promotes clarity.
3. Ujjayi (Victorious Breath): Often used in asana practice, ujjayi is a soft, whispering breath that deepens the connection between body and mind, enhancing focus and concentration.
4. Kapalbhati (Skull Shining Breath): A quick, forceful exhalation technique that detoxifies the body and clears mental fog, leaving you refreshed.

5. **Bhramari (Bee Breath):** A soothing breath that involves a gentle humming sound, calming the nervous system and reducing anxiety.

With regular breath work and consistent practice, I've built up the stamina to incorporate different forms of yoga into my routine, including power yoga. Power yoga is a more intense form of yoga that combines strength and cardio, challenging both the body and the mind. It's the perfect blend of endurance and mindfulness, and I love the way it keeps my body engaged while helping me stay mentally focused.

If you're new to yoga, I recommend starting small. Begin with 10 rounds of Surya Namaskar. Add some stretching, include a few pranayama exercises, and focus on your breath. These small steps will bring a sense of calm and clarity. Start slow, and over time, you'll find your stamina building. Soon enough, you'll be able to do 50, 100, or even 108 Surya Namaskars, just like we do in an intense class. Yoga, for me, is about consistency, building strength, and, most important, listening to my body.

My Yoga Routine: Asanas and Postures

As yoga became an integral part of my fitness journey, I started to tailor my routine to suit my needs and goals. Here are a few asanas that I practise regularly, each with its own unique benefits for both my body and my mind.

Surya Namaskar (Sun Salutation)

As mentioned earlier, Surya Namaskar has been a staple in my daily practice for years now. I start every single day with it. Not only does it serve as a perfect cardio workout, but it is also a spiritual and mental cleanse that helps me connect with my body and breath. For me, it's a complete body workout that boosts my metabolism, tones muscles, and stretches every part of my body. It's a practice that keeps me grounded both physically and mentally. Here's a closer look at how I approach it.

Step-by-Step Guide
1. **Pranamasana (Prayer Pose):** Start by standing tall, feet together, and palms pressed together in prayer at your chest.
2. **Hasta Uttanasana (Raised Arms Pose):** Inhale and raise your arms overhead, slightly arching your back.
3. **Padahastasana (Hand to Foot Pose):** Exhale and fold forward, bringing your hands to the floor beside your feet.

4. **Ashwa Sanchalanasana (Equestrian Pose):** Step your right leg back and bring your chest forward, lifting your gaze.
5. **Dandasana (Stick Pose):** Step back into plank position, keeping your body straight.
6. **Ashtanga Namaskara (Salute with Eight Limbs):** Lower your knees, chest, and chin to the floor, keeping your hips up.
7. **Bhujangasana (Cobra Pose):** Inhale and lift your chest, bending your spine upward, supported by your hands.
8. **Adho Mukha Svanasana (Downward Facing Dog):** Exhale and lift your hips up and back, forming an inverted V-shape with your body.
9. **Ashwa Sanchalanasana:** Step your right foot forward, keeping your chest lifted.
10. **Padahastasana:** Step your left foot forward, bringing both feet together.
11. **Hasta Uttanasana:** Inhale and rise to a standing position, your arms raised overhead, back slightly arched.
12. **Pranamasana:** Exhale and return to the starting position.

Parivrtta Trikonasana (Revolved Triangle Pose)

This pose is a great way to open up the hips, lengthen the spine, and improve balance. It also helps to engage the core and strengthens the legs.

Steps
1. Begin with feet wide apart, right foot facing out and left foot slightly turned in.
2. Inhale and extend your arms out to the sides.
3. Exhale and rotate your torso to the right, bringing your left hand to your right foot while extending your right arm upward.
4. Keep your legs strong and engage your core to hold the position.

Benefits: Strengthens the legs, opens the hips, and increases spinal flexibility.

Ashwa Sanchalanasana (Equestrian Pose)

This is a perfect pose for stretching the hip flexors and building strength in the legs and lower back.

Steps
1. From Downward Dog, step your right foot forward between your hands.
2. Lower your left knee to the ground and raise your arms overhead.
3. Relax your shoulders and look up, deepening the stretch.

Benefits: Stretches the hip flexors, strengthens the legs, and opens the chest.

Adho Mukha Svanasana (Downward Facing Dog)

A classic yoga pose that is great for stretching the back, strengthening the arms, and calming the mind.

Steps
1. Start on all fours and lift your hips towards the ceiling, straightening your legs and arms.
2. Press your heels towards the floor while keeping your back straight and head between your arms.

Benefits: Stretches the back, tones the core, and strengthens the arms and legs.

Natarajasana (Dancer's Pose)

This balancing pose is excellent for improving posture, flexibility, and balance.

Steps
1. Stand on your left leg, bend your right knee and grab your right ankle with your right hand.
2. Extend your left arm forward and kick your right leg back.
3. Keep your chest lifted and try to balance while stretching.

Benefits: Improves balance, strengthens the back, and stretches the legs and chest.

Utthita Hasta Padangusthasana (Extended Hand-to-Big-Toe Pose)

A wonderful pose for balance and core strength, while also stretching the legs.

Steps
1. Stand tall and lift your right leg, holding your big toe with your right hand.
2. Extend the leg forward, to the side, or even behind you, depending on your flexibility.

Benefits: Improves balance, strengthens the core, and stretches the hamstrings.

Sarvangasana (Shoulder Stand)

This inversion helps stimulate the thyroid, improves circulation, and calms the nervous system.

Steps
1. Lie on your back and lift your legs overhead, supporting your back with your hands.
2. Keep your legs straight and perpendicular to the floor.
3. Hold the position for a few breaths, maintaining stability and control.

Benefits: Improves circulation, strengthens the shoulders, and relieves stress.

There are many more asanas, each serving a unique purpose – whether it's backbends, tree pose, or butterfly pose. I could go on and on. Some work wonders for the back, others target the stomach, and there are poses that help with things like thyroid issues or dry eyes. I remember how poses like the fish pose helped me when I was struggling with dry eyes. The beauty of yoga is that you don't have to commit to it exclusively – you can blend it with any other workout. It's something I swear by and highly recommend for overall health and well-being.

Neti: A Sacred Part of My Wellness Routine

Neti, a traditional yogic practice, plays an essential role in my daily wellness rituals. It's a form of nasal irrigation that helps me clear my sinuses, improve my breathing, and enhance my mental clarity. There are two types of Neti that I practise: Jal Neti and Vaman Neti.

- Jal Neti involves using saline water to flush the nasal passages. It's a soothing, cleansing practice that rejuvenates both the body and mind.

- Vaman Neti, on the other hand, is a deeper cleanse that I perform occasionally when I feel I need a more intense internal reset.

The reason I incorporate Neti into my routine is simple: with constant travel, long hours, and being on the go, Neti helps me ensure I'm not only physically healthy but mentally sharp. It's a wonderful way to alleviate stress, maintain mental clarity, and support my body's natural rhythm.

Steps to Perform Jal Neti (Nasal Irrigation)
1. Prepare your Neti pot and saline solution (1 teaspoon of salt per cup of warm, distilled water).
2. Tilt your head to one side over a sink, keeping your chin slightly tucked in.
3. Gently pour the saline solution into one nostril. Allow the water to flow through and out the other nostril.
4. Breathe through your mouth during the process.
5. Repeat on the other side.
6. Gently blow your nose to clear any remaining water.

When to Perform Neti
I usually perform Neti in the morning, just after waking up, before starting my yoga or workout routine. It's an

excellent way to clear any mucus from the night and prepare my body for the day ahead. I typically practise it two to three times a week, depending on how my body feels. Overdoing it can lead to dryness or irritation, so it's important to listen to your body.

Benefits of Neti

- Improved Breathing: Neti clears the nasal passages, making breathing easier.
- Mental Clarity: It helps clear mental fog, preparing me to tackle the day with focus and energy.
- Prevention of Sinus Infections: Regular practice reduces the risk of sinus infections by preventing the build-up of mucus and irritants.
- Grounding: The cleansing ritual of Neti provides a calming, grounding effect, essential for my busy lifestyle.

Diva Yoga Studio: The Heart of My Practice

After years of personal transformation through yoga, I felt called to share that journey with others. And that's how Diva Yoga Studio came into being. It's more than just a studio – it's a sanctuary, a space where women (and men, of course) can come together to connect with their bodies, nurture their minds, and discover the power of yoga in their own lives. I've always believed in yoga's potential to heal, strengthen, and bring balance, and I wanted to create a space where others could experience the same transformation.

The Philosophy Behind Diva Yoga Studio

At Diva Yoga, we offer a variety of yoga styles to cater to different needs. From Vinyasa for fluid movement and flow, to Hatha for more gentle, restorative practice, and power yoga for those looking for an intense workout – there is something for everyone. The aim is to provide a well-rounded approach to fitness, combining both physical strength and mental clarity. I've seen how yoga has completely changed my life, and I want to offer others the same opportunity to find balance, strength, and peace.

When I created Diva Yoga, I wanted it to be a space free of judgement, where people could practise yoga at their own pace. Whether you're a beginner or an experienced yogi, Diva Yoga is meant to be a welcoming space where you can fully embrace your yoga journey.

Sharing the Yoga Journey

One of the things I'm most passionate about is spreading the message of yoga to as many people as possible. That's why I've made it a point to share the teachings and practices of Diva Yoga through Instagram (@thedivayoga). Whether it's posting short workout routines, breathing exercises, or motivational tips, I want to inspire others to adopt yoga as part of their daily lives. We also share snippets from our classes and encourage people to join us in our community of wellness.

Yoga is meant to be shared. I believe that if you can transform yourself through yoga, you can help transform the world around you.

Pilates: Enhancing Core Strength and Flexibility

While yoga has always been the foundation of my routine, Pilates brings a complementary element that I absolutely swear by. It's not just a workout; it's a system that promotes controlled, precise movements that focus on strengthening the core, improving flexibility, and enhancing overall body alignment. Pilates has become indispensable for injury prevention and posture correction. It's not just about toning muscles, it's about cultivating awareness of the body and its movements.

My Pilates Journey: The Power of Control and Precision

When I first began practising Pilates, I wasn't sure how it would fit into my routine. I had always been more inclined towards high-intensity workouts or yoga.

However, after a few sessions, I quickly realized that Pilates offered something entirely different. Under the expert guidance of my trainer, Namrata Purohit, I learned to embrace slow, controlled movements that allowed me to strengthen my core without the risk of injury. As a result, my balance improved, and I developed a much deeper understanding of how my body moves in space. Pilates helped me recover from injuries and restored stability to my body.

I especially love the core-focused exercises because they have a direct impact on my posture and overall strength. I often train with a friend or a buddy, as it makes the sessions so much more fun. Pilates is about engaging the deeper muscles that aren't always targeted by traditional workouts. It's about creating strength from the inside out, and I've found that this focus on the core has had a positive effect on my yoga practice and in my daily life.

Key Pilates Exercises I Love

Here are some of the exercises I love incorporating into my routine:

The Saw
Sit with your legs extended wide apart and your arms outstretched at shoulder height. Inhale and lengthen

your spine, then twist your torso to the right. Reach your left hand towards your right foot while keeping your legs grounded. Return to the centre and repeat on the other side.

Variation: On some days, I deepen the twist or slow down the movement to really engage the obliques and work on spinal flexibility. These small adjustments help target different areas and keep the routine dynamic.

Benefits: This exercise improves spinal mobility, stretches the back and hamstrings, strengthens the core, and enhances posture and alignment.

Leg Circles

Lie on your back with one leg extended towards the ceiling. Keep your hips stable as you make small, controlled circles with your leg. Gradually increase the size of the circles, then reverse the direction after several repetitions.

Benefits: This targets the hip flexors, improves joint mobility, and helps in strengthening the lower body, particularly the thighs and hips.

Pilates Push-Ups

Start in a standing position and slowly roll down to a plank. Perform a push-up, engaging your core, then roll back up to standing.

Benefits: Combines upper body strength and core stability. It's an amazing way to work both your arms and your core, providing a full-body challenge.

Bridges

Lie on your back with knees bent and feet flat on the floor. Lift your hips towards the ceiling, squeezing your glutes and engaging your core. Hold for a moment at the top and then lower back down.

Benefits: Bridges target the glutes and lower back, improving lower body strength and posture.

Weight Training: Building Strength and Endurance

Weight training really transformed my body. It's essential for developing strength, toning muscles, and improving the body's metabolic rate. I felt everything tighten up – my body became more defined, with less jiggle, and the strength was unmistakable – something that only comes with weight training. When I combined that with yoga, it felt like the perfect match! While I love Pilates and yoga, weight training ensures that my body has the muscle mass it needs for functional strength and longevity.

Why Weight Training Is Key to My Fitness Routine

Weight training plays a pivotal role in shaping and maintaining my body. It's not about bulking up, but rather toning and maintaining a lean, strong physique. Over the years, I've learned that weight training not only helps build muscle but also enhances my endurance, making me more resilient in all areas of my life – from carrying groceries to holding a yoga pose for longer periods. It's also crucial for maintaining bone density, especially as I age, and reducing the risk of injury.

Incorporating weight training with yoga and Pilates ensures a holistic approach to fitness. Yoga gives me flexibility and mental clarity, Pilates strengthens the core, and weight training builds muscle strength that supports both. Together, they create a well-rounded routine that works every part of my body.

Effective Weight Training Exercises

Here are some of the key weight training exercises I include in my routine:

Squats

Stand with your feet shoulder-width apart and toes slightly pointed outward. Push your hips back and lower your body as if you are sitting in a chair. Keep your back straight and knees behind your toes. Return to standing.

Benefits: Squats are an excellent lower-body exercise, targeting the quads, hamstrings, and glutes. They also engage your core and improve mobility and flexibility.

Chest Press

Lie on a bench with a dumbbell in each hand. Start with the weights at shoulder level, elbows bent. Press the weights upward until your arms are fully extended, then lower them back down slowly.

Benefits: This exercise targets the chest, shoulders, and triceps, helping to build upper-body strength and endurance.

Deadlifts

Stand with feet hip-width apart, holding a barbell in front of your thighs. Keeping your back straight, hinge at the hips, lowering the barbell down the front of your legs, then return to standing.

Benefits: Deadlifts are fantastic for strengthening the posterior chain, including the back, hamstrings, glutes, and core. This compound movement builds functional strength and improves posture.

Tricep Dips

Place your hands on a bench or platform behind you, legs extended forward. Lower your body down by bending your elbows, keeping your back close to the bench. Push yourself back up to the starting position.

Benefits: This exercise targets the triceps, shoulders, and chest, helping tone and strengthen the upper body.

Bicep Curls

Stand with your feet shoulder-width apart, holding a dumbbell in each hand. Curl the weights towards your shoulders, keeping your elbows close to your body. Slowly lower the weights back down.

Benefits: Bicep curls are an excellent exercise for building strength in the arms and forearms, contributing to overall arm definition.

Weekly Exercise Routine Breakdown

Day	Exercise Focus	Details
Monday	Lower Body + Yoga	Weight training for legs using free weights (no machines), followed by a yoga stretch session to relax the muscles
Tuesday	Upper Body + Cardio	Weight training for arms and shoulders using free weights, followed by a 20-minute run for cardio

Day	Exercise Focus	Details
Wednesday	Yoga + Pilates (Core Focus)	Focus on Pilates for core strength and yoga for flexibility, possibly using light ankle weights during yoga for added resistance
Thursday	Full Body Weight Training + Yoga	Strength training for all body parts using free weights, followed by a calming yoga session to ease the lactic acid build-up and promote flexibility
Friday	Cardio + Stretching	30 minutes of brisk walking followed by deep stretching to maintain flexibility and reduce stress
Saturday	Traditional Yoga + Stretching	Focus on deep traditional yoga stretches, incorporating TRX stretching and emphasizing flexibility and muscle relaxation
Sunday	Rest Day / Light Activity	Light walking or restorative yoga for recovery, providing the body with much-needed relaxation and mental clarity

Mindfulness Through Movement

Fitness has become my sanctuary. It's where I go when I need to clear my mind, calm my nerves, or fight anxiety. As much as fitness has transformed my body, the real change came mentally. Fitness has become a tool not just for physical transformation but for emotional healing as well. Every day, whether it's yoga, a quick walk, or just some time to meditate, I take that moment for myself. It's what keeps me grounded, and helps me navigate daily stress while maintaining a positive mindset. Yoga, especially, has had a transformative impact on my mental clarity.

There was a time when work pressure was mounting, and I was dealing with personal challenges. Yoga became my emotional reset button. It was during this time that I truly leaned into pranayama – the deep breathing that brought peace back into my chaotic mind. Since then, I've prioritized mindfulness and breath work in my daily routine. It's a practice I can't recommend enough for anyone trying to find mental balance in a hectic world.

I love walking. It's simple, effective, gives me that moment of calm, and doesn't require fancy equipment or a gym. Whether I'm in the middle of a busy shoot or on the move while travelling, just 30 minutes of walking can clear my head. It keeps my heart strong, boosts circulation, and improves cognitive function. Walking is one of those underrated exercises that not only keeps the body healthy but helps the mind stay clear too. There's something meditative about it. When I walk, I tune in to my surroundings, focus on my breath, or sometimes even recite a mantra. It's my go-to for de-stressing, especially when life gets overwhelming.

Once when I was experiencing a mental fog, barely sleeping, and feeling drained, I decided to step outside for a quick 20-minute walk around the block. As soon as I did, everything shifted – the fresh air, the rhythmic movement, and the space to think clearly. That walk became my reset button. It's been a reliable tool for mental clarity ever since.

I'm more resilient today and mentally stronger, and whenever stress tries to take over, I turn to movement for clarity. These practices provide me with emotional stability and a sense of peace, no matter what life throws my way.

A Love Affair with Movement (and Yourself)

I won't sugarcoat it: there are days when I'm running on an empty tank. I may be dog-tired after a long night or just unable to kick myself out of bed early in the morning, and the last thing I want to do is work out.

There are times when I think, 'One more hour of sleep might do me good.' But I've learned over time that it's in those moments, when my brain is negotiating with me, that I need to remind myself why I started this journey in the first place. I remind myself that the benefits of showing up and committing to my routine are always greater than the temporary relief of a few extra minutes in bed.

Motivation doesn't always come easily: you have to create it. I've learned to treat fitness like a love affair with myself. On tough days, when I'm drained or tempted to skip my workout, I remind myself that I'm strong, capable, and worth the effort. That internal validation powers me through the dips. You can't wait for motivation to strike; you've got to build it from within.

Over time, I've come to realize that consistency and discipline are everything. It's the small, everyday choices that become long-term investments in your well-being. Fitness is about balance, not perfection – and definitely not about logging endless hours at the gym. When I say I make time for fitness, I don't mean I'm running myself into the ground. I've learned that listening to my body is just as important as sticking to a routine. If I'm truly exhausted, I rest. Rest is not failure; it's recovery. Some days will be harder than others, and self-compassion is vital. I've learned not to beat myself up for needing a break.

There are also days when I know I need to push through, and I do. The goal is balance: staying active without overwhelming my body. I mix things up. Sometimes it's yoga, other times Pilates or a walk. On high-energy days, I go all out. On others, I take it easy with a gentler routine. The point is to stay consistent. That's what builds fitness over time. It's not about the extremes; it's about showing up, again and again.

When I was younger, fitness was about intensity: jumping from one workout to the next without truly listening to what my body needed. But now I know better. It's not about pushing your limits every day. It's about creating a steady, sustainable habit – one that evolves with your needs, your age, your energy levels. That's what makes fitness a lifestyle.

Of course, social media can make it hard. We're often bombarded with intense workouts and unrealistic body standards. But that's not real life. You don't need to run marathons or lift heavy weights to stay fit. Even something as simple as a 15-minute walk daily can work wonders for your physical and mental health. What matters most is showing up, consistently and mindfully.

And if you're doing everything right but not seeing results, don't give up. Sometimes, your body might be telling you it needs a deeper check-in. For me, getting certain health markers tested helped uncover internal issues that needed attention. Once I addressed them, the results followed. So don't be afraid to listen closely and investigate.

This mindset and discipline have helped me stay fit through the years, even while juggling shoots, travel, and everything life throws at me. Sometimes, you have to say no to other things to say yes to yourself. That's how I've kept going – not through perfection, but through presence and commitment.

The Wellness Puzzle: Sleep, Nutrition, and Fitness

Fitness isn't a standalone achievement. It only works when it's supported by everything else we've already talked about: sleep, rest, and food that nourishes you. Trust me when I tell you that you could put in all the effort at the gym, but if your body isn't well rested or well fuelled, you'll hit a wall. No movement plan, no matter how consistent, can make up for poor sleep or neglectful eating.

Sleep is where the magic happens. It's the time when your body repairs, your muscles recover, and your hormones reset. Without it, I feel foggy, drained, and disconnected from my workouts. That's why rest has become a non-negotiable part of my routine. As I've said before, true glow doesn't come from products – it comes from how well you sleep, eat, and move. Nutrition is just as essential. I've already spoken about how I eat for energy, for my skin, and for balance – not to chase a trend. That same food fuels my workouts and helps my body bounce back. When I started seeing food as nourishment and sleep as recovery, everything shifted. I wasn't just exercising – I was thriving.

For me, that's the real puzzle of wellness: aligning sleep, nutrition, and fitness so they support each other. That's when the body responds, the energy flows, and the results last. Anything less, and it's just noise.

Desk Stretches and Posture: Simple Steps for a Healthier You

Now many of us lead sedentary lifestyles – whether it's due to desk jobs, long hours spent in front of screens, or just general busyness. I understand how challenging it can be to squeeze fitness into a hectic schedule. But even if you can't make it to the gym, that doesn't mean you're doomed to aches and stiffness! It's about taking small steps to keep your body moving, no matter how busy you are.

I often hear from friends who struggle with posture issues, neck pain, or back stiffness due to sitting for long hours. The good news is it doesn't take a lot to protect yourself from these common pains. A few simple stretches and being mindful of your posture can make a huge difference. I always encourage those with desk jobs to take a minute every few hours to do a simple stretch or move around. These small actions can prevent long-term discomfort and boost your energy.

Desk Stretches I Recommend

These desk stretches will help release tension and keep your body in good shape.
- **Restorative Forward Bend:** Sit at the edge of your chair with feet flat on the floor. Gently bend forward and let your chest rest towards your thighs. This stretch releases back tension and calms the mind.
- **The Wrist Stretch:** Extend your arm forward with your palm facing up, then gently pull your fingers back to stretch your forearms and wrists. Perfect if you're typing for long hours.

Fitness: More Than Just a Look

- **Chest Opener:** Sit up tall, place your hands on the armrests, and push your chest forward while rolling your shoulders back. This helps counteract the hunching posture that often comes from sitting too long.
- **Neck Extensions:** Slowly roll your head in a circular motion to release neck stiffness. Keep it gentle to avoid strain.

The key to managing a sedentary lifestyle is not striving for perfection, but consistency. Even if you can only fit in 10-minute sessions throughout your day, just moving and stretching regularly will keep you flexible and energized. Aiming for 5,000 steps a day is a great goal to start with. Whether it's a walk on your lunch break or simply getting up to stretch every hour, every little bit counts. Ayurveda recommends a very short brisk walk after each meal for gut health. I've personally seen its effects on friends who suffer from GERD and IBS. It makes the indigestion and bloating so much more manageable.

As for posture, it's something I keep hearing about from friends, especially those working long hours at a desk. Many people don't realize how important it is to maintain a neutral spine throughout the day. Poor posture can lead to neck pain, back issues, and even headaches. Yoga has taught me the importance of spine health, and the best way to protect your body is by keeping everything aligned – your head, neck, and spine. A small adjustment like sitting with your feet flat on the floor, shoulders relaxed, and your ears in line with your shoulders can go a long way. I also make sure to move around regularly throughout the day, even if it's just for a minute or two.

Incorporating these simple stretches and being mindful of your posture can help protect your body from the aches, pains, and lifestyle diseases that often come with sitting too long. The more consistent you are, the better you'll feel.

Final Word: Fitness as Self-Care

Fitness isn't just about looking good; it's about feeling good, inside and out. The real transformation happens when fitness becomes part of your lifestyle – a daily investment in your health. It's not about pushing yourself to extremes but about making time for movement that supports your mind and body. Whether it's yoga, a brisk walk, or a quick workout, consistency and balance are key.

For me, fitness is my moment of self-care. It grounds me, keeps me centred, and helps me stay at my best amid life's demands. Whether it's stepping on the mat for yoga, lifting weights, or doing a simple stretch, I've learned that showing up for yourself, day after day, is what truly builds strength.

Your fitness journey doesn't have to be extreme to be effective. It's about tuning in to your body and finding joy in the process. When you prioritize your wellness, the rewards ripple across every part of your life. So stay consistent, be kind to yourself, and keep moving forward – one step, one stretch, one breath at a time.

6

Women's Health:
Navigating the Phases of Life

As women, we're constantly told what we should be at every stage of our lives. The expectations can feel relentless, especially as we age. Words like 'divorcee' and 'too old' get thrown around on my socials, as if turning 50 means fading into the background. But I'm living proof that age is just a number. I feel more confident, independent, and alive than ever. I'm still making people shake a leg with my songs, running my own businesses, and living life on my own terms.

From the energy-filled days of my twenties to the emotional and physical shifts of pregnancy, postpartum, and now perimenopause, I've experienced it all. There were moments when I didn't recognize my own body or felt unsure of who I was becoming. But with time, I've learned to embrace each phase with curiosity, compassion, and grace. The key is listening – to your body, your emotions, your energy – and adjusting with care instead of resistance.

And here's the truth: even with all the work I put into my routines — eating right, staying active, being consistent — there are days I still feel off. That's the paradox of being a woman. You can do everything 'right' and still have your body surprise you. Hormonal shifts, mood swings, unexplained fatigue. It's a constant dance. And unfortunately, medical science still hasn't fully caught up with our lived experiences. So we keep figuring it out, often on our own. That's what's made me kinder to myself and more determined to keep learning.

This chapter is an honest reflection of that journey, from physical transformation to emotional growth. I'm not here to prescribe, only to share what's helped me navigate the ups and downs of womanhood. Because no matter where you are in your journey, you deserve to feel seen, supported, and strong in your body. If I can do it, so can you.

Laying the Foundation for Life in Your Twenties

Your twenties are a time of exploration. It's when you begin discovering who you are, what matters to you, and how to navigate life's many changes. It's also a crucial phase for laying the groundwork for a healthier, more balanced future. For me, those years were all about self-discovery, learning to nourish my body, and figuring out how to prioritize physical and mental health, even when it felt like there wasn't enough time to pause.

Back then, I was constantly on the move, juggling work, dance, and everything else life threw my way. Fitness was part of it, though I didn't think about it quite the way I do today. It was more about staying in shape for my career, working out for stamina and aesthetics, while keeping up with a demanding schedule. But as I mentioned in the previous chapter, those routines, even when rooted in discipline and performance, planted the seeds of something deeper: a more mindful, long-term relationship with movement.

Dance, especially, shaped this phase of my life. It wasn't just movement – it was empowerment. I felt alive in my body. Even though I didn't have a formal wellness mindset yet, dance taught me discipline, boosted my confidence, and, although unplanned, set the tone for the lifestyle I'd build later. In hindsight, this was my body's early way of telling me what it needed. That's something I've become much more attuned to over the years, especially through yoga and strength work.

Looking back now, I can see how vital it was to find balance, not just between work and workouts, but between movement and rest, hustle and self-care. In my mid-twenties, I started realizing that real strength came from tuning in, not pushing through. That shift in mindset was everything. Fitness became about more than just looking good. It became about feeling grounded, strong, and whole. That's the perspective that still guides me: wellness as a lifelong practice of balance, nourishment, and self-awareness.

> For Women in Their Twenties: Start simple. Build habits that nourish your body and calm your mind. The choices you make now become the foundation for your future health, and trust me, they're worth it.

Pregnancy and Postpartum: Embracing Transformation

I've spoken before about how motherhood changed me – physically, mentally, and emotionally – but it deserves its own space here, because becoming a mother in my late twenties was one of the most transformative experiences of my life. Pregnancy, for me, wasn't just a physical change. It was a deep, ongoing journey that touched every part of me. While I had always been active and involved in fitness, pregnancy challenged my body in ways I hadn't anticipated. Cultivating self-care and learning to listen to my body became more important than ever. I stayed active throughout:

daily walks, pregnancy yoga, and tuning in to what my body needed. However, I didn't push myself too hard. The focus was on staying connected with my body, not striving for perfection.

During this time, I also learned to embrace moderation. It's easy to fall for the old myth that you're 'eating for two', something I touched on in the food chapter. But even then, I chose a more mindful approach – satisfying cravings without losing sight of balance. That mindset, built over years of tuning in to my body, helped me stay healthy and active through pregnancy, which made the postpartum recovery a little smoother. Walking daily and attending prenatal classes became anchors in my routine.

Postpartum, however, brought a different kind of challenge. I found myself facing the pressure of returning to my pre-pregnancy body – a societal expectation so many women encounter after childbirth. I remember staring at my reflection in disbelief, feeling disconnected and uncertain about how to navigate the changes. Stretch marks, a new body shape ... it was a lot to process emotionally. There were moments when I seriously considered surgical options to 'fix' what I saw as 'imperfections'. But over time, I chose patience. I reminded myself of something I've said before: wellness is a journey, not a race.

It took about three months before I began to see any change. During this time, I focused on gentle stretches and walks and slowly brought yoga back into my life. These were tools I'd leaned on for years. I didn't rush it. I wasn't trying to 'bounce back', nor did I expect to look exactly the same. This was a new version of me, and I had to meet her with grace.

Still, I won't pretend it was easy. I was deeply upset every time I looked in the mirror. The weight was hanging in places that felt unfamiliar. My stomach no longer looked like mine, and I kept asking myself: How did this happen? I had always been so disciplined, so conscious about my health and fitness. And yet, this new body felt like it belonged to someone else. I would cry – not because of the stretch marks, but because I couldn't recognize the person staring back. It was as if I'd been through a battle and come out changed in ways I wasn't prepared for. The pressure to 'bounce back' was suffocating. But slowly, I reminded myself of what I already knew. I wasn't supposed to look the same. My body had done something extraordinary. It deserved time and respect.

One of the biggest lessons I learned during this period was patience – not the passive kind, but the active, compassionate kind. It wasn't about going back to 'normal'. It was about discovering a new normal. I didn't want to obsess over weight loss. I didn't want to be defined by this change. I had to respect the process.

Eventually, I turned to weight training. I've spoken about this in the chapter on fitness too, but it truly became the game changer for me post-pregnancy. It wasn't about shedding kilos. It was about rebuilding strength. Weight training helped me reconnect with my body. I began to feel stronger, more stable, and more like myself. My muscles felt engaged again. That loose, jiggly feeling started to fade, replaced by a growing sense of definition and control – mentally and physically.

When I added yoga back into the mix, everything clicked. Yoga, with its stretches, breathing, and introspection, complemented the strength and structure of weight training. Together, they brought me back to a place of balance. It was a place I hadn't been in for a long time.

I'd be lying if I said I've made peace with everything. There are still days when I look at my lower belly and wish I could smooth it all out. I still hesitate to show my stomach. I'm still conscious of my stretch marks. But when people troll me for it – and yes, they do – I just think: these are my battle scars. I've birthed a child. This body tells a story. It's taken time, but I've come to accept that this version of me deserves love too.

> **For Women in Postpartum:** Take your time. There's no rush to get back to your pre-pregnancy body. Focus on recovery, self-compassion, and gradual progress. Your body is your guide – trust it.

Perimenopause: A Phase of Change and Understanding

Perimenopause – a word that wasn't even in my vocabulary until just a few years ago. I'm sure it's the same for many women, especially in our culture. We talk about menopause, but rarely do we discuss the years leading up to it – the time when hormonal changes begin, but we don't yet understand exactly what's happening in our bodies. I found myself in that place not long ago when, during a routine check-up, my doctor told me I was entering perimenopause, even though I hadn't yet felt its full impact.

A lot of it comes down to the lifestyle I've cultivated over the years – regular check-ups, balanced nutrition, movement, and sleep. I've emphasized this time and again throughout this book, and now I see just how much those choices have helped. My commitment to wellness has undoubtedly delayed the symptoms that many women experience. I've always been particular about my habits: eating clean, staying active, and prioritizing rest. But even with those long-standing practices, I'm not immune to the changes this phase brings. At 49, I can feel the shifts in my body. My sleep patterns are no longer as restful, and I've started experiencing mood swings that can be intense. While I haven't yet had hot flashes, I know many women who are battling them fiercely. For some, perimenopause is seamless; for others, it's much more turbulent. What matters is acknowledging that this phase is real – and that we need to talk about it more openly.

Perimenopause isn't something we should brush under the rug. There's still so little awareness, and we often don't give ourselves permission to talk about it or seek help. But it's essential to understand that this transition is both common and manageable – especially when you're informed and proactive. As with other stages I've experienced – pregnancy, postpartum, emotional shifts – I've learned that we can't afford to live passively. We need to respond with the same mindset I've always championed: awareness, acceptance, and action. You have to accept the emotional and physical shifts and adapt. It's not about striving for the body you had in your twenties or thirties. It's about feeling strong, flexible, and at peace with where you are. I'm determined to keep living fully, without letting these changes hold me back. Embrace these transitions. Take care of your body, nourish your mind, and stay active. There's no stopping you.

Tackling the Challenges of Perimenopause

There's no magic cure for perimenopause, but there are lifestyle adjustments that can make this transition easier. As I approach 50, I've started tweaking my habits – much like I've done through other big shifts in my life – to make this phase a little easier to manage. While it's inevitable, there's a lot you can do to ease the journey.

> ### Lifestyle Tweaks for Managing Perimenopause
> - **Stay Active:** Exercise – whether it's yoga, walking, or strength training – continues to be one of my biggest allies. As I shared earlier in the chapter on fitness, movement has always helped regulate not just my body but my mind. It plays a huge role in managing hormonal fluctuations and the emotional roller coaster that perimenopause can be. Staying active helps balance out the changes happening in my body. It doesn't just keep my weight in check – it helps stabilize mood swings, boosts energy, and gives me the strength I need to take on each day.

- **Support System:** Perimenopause doesn't only affect you; it impacts everyone around you. For many women, mood swings can be overwhelming, and it can affect your relationships and work life. Having a support system – friends, family, or a partner who understands – can make a world of difference. I've said this before and I'll say it again: healing and wellness are rarely solo journeys. The people around you matter. Don't forget to communicate with them.

  Perimenopause is a time to take charge of your health, so don't hesitate to get expert advice. Make sure to consult your doctor for a personalized approach to supplements, diet, and exercise.

- **Be Gentle with Yourself:** I've learned that perimenopause can stir up emotional ups and downs, and sometimes I feel I'm losing control of my body and emotions. But I've come to accept that this is part of the process. When I noticed changes in my body, I didn't try to fight them. I focused on managing what I could: staying active, eating well, and allowing myself grace. I even started taking certain vitamins recommended by my doctor to replenish what

my body was losing during this time. Some days, I feel bloated, sluggish, and emotional – and that's OK. I give myself the space to feel what I feel without judgement. That mindset – of self-compassion, not perfection – is one I've cultivated since my twenties. These phases are temporary and manageable with the right mindset.
- **Embrace Change:** One of the biggest lessons I've learned is to embrace perimenopause as a new chapter, not an obstacle. I refuse to let this phase dictate how I live my life. I'm still exploring, still travelling, still enjoying the things I love. Age is not a limitation. If anything, it can be a gateway to new kinds of strength. I truly believe what I've said many times before: taking care of yourself – physically, mentally, emotionally – is never a phase. It's a commitment, and one that evolves with you. There's freedom in this stage of life if you allow yourself to see it.

Menopause: A New Beginning, Not an End

When we talk about menopause, many women think it's the end of something – the end of youth, end of vitality. But that's not the case. Menopause, for me, was more like the beginning of a new chapter. Yes, your body will change. Yes, your sexual drive might decrease. You may no longer be able to reproduce, and your hormones will fluctuate. But none of that means your life is over. It's simply the start of a different kind of freedom.

I've heard from many women that post-50, they're living their best lives. And I believe it. It's not about clinging to the past or fearing what lies ahead – it's about embracing change, something I've had to learn through every phase, whether it was pregnancy, postpartum, or perimenopause. We've been conditioned to fear menopause or tiptoe around it as if it's something shameful. But I'm here to tell you: don't fear it. This is a time for liberation. You can still love, connect, travel, explore – life doesn't stop after 50. In fact, it can become more vibrant than ever.

Rituals for Every Phase of Life

What's helped me most through all these transitions – whether it was the energy of my twenties, the shifts in my thirties, or the reflection of my forties – has been building routines that support where I'm at. Not rigid ones, but flexible, sustainable habits that evolve with me. I've never believed in extreme diets or punishing workouts. I simply listen to my body, and adjust as needed.

> ### Rituals I Come Back To
>
> - **Morning Stretch:** A quick yoga flow or gentle stretching to ease into the day.
> - **Strength Training:** A mix of weights and bodyweight movements to build and maintain strength.
> - **Rest Days:** Either a long walk or deep stretching – anything that helps me recharge.
> - **Self-Care:** Whether it's journaling, meditation, or quiet time, I carve out space to care for my mind just as much as my body.

Each phase brings its own needs, and the most important thing I've learned is to move in sync with them. Consistency – not intensity – is what keeps me grounded.

The Importance of Regular Check-Ups: Taking Control of Your Health

Now let's talk about something that doesn't get enough attention: regular check-ups. Women are so often conditioned to prioritize everyone else – families, careers, relationships – that we sometimes forget to look after ourselves. But our bodies are our responsibility. And regular health check-ups are one of the most powerful ways to take that responsibility seriously, especially as we grow older.

For me, that lesson came into sharp focus when I was diagnosed with uterine polyps in my thirties. I had them removed, but they returned more than once, each time reminding me that ignoring my health wasn't an option. Polyps are usually benign, but if left unchecked, they can cause complications with menstruation and even fertility. Staying on top of regular scans and doctor visits helped me avoid bigger issues and gave me peace of mind.

Around the same time, I also began noticing changes in my skin – hyperpigmentation, dullness, and patches that didn't look or feel familiar. That's when I decided to see a dermatologist. They recommended a few options, including topical retinol and medicated creams tailored to my needs. But what helped most wasn't a single product; it was the mindset of adapting my skincare routine to fit my changing body. I still enjoy home remedies and natural solutions, but now I balance them with products that support ageing skin. For example, serums became a staple in my forties. Earlier, my skin didn't need that extra boost, but as the years passed, I leaned into products that could nourish it more deeply.

Another check-up I never skip is the mammogram. I'll admit, they're not the most pleasant experience, but after the age of 40, they become essential. Thankfully, newer technologies like 3D mammograms have made the process more comfortable. Alongside professional screenings, I also do regular self-exams. It's simple: check for any lumps, hard knots, or unusual changes in texture or size. A few minutes in front of the mirror or in the shower can make a huge difference. And if you're unsure how to go about it, ask your gynaecologist at your next visit. They'll walk you through it without judgement, so don't feel awkward or shy.

Of course, check-ups aren't just about what you can see or feel. Hormonal shifts can impact your mood, sleep, energy, and sense of self. I've touched on this earlier while discussing perimenopause and menopause, but no matter your age, being in tune with your health is empowering. I now make it a point to get regular blood work done and check in with my doctor about my nutrient levels. Knowing where I stand helps me feel more in control.

Relying on supplements based on my body's needs, especially as I navigate this new phase of life, is something I have talked about at length in the chapter on food. Some were recommended by my doctor, like B-complex, calcium, magnesium, and vitamin D. Collagen has become another focus, particularly after 40, when the body's natural production starts to slow. I usually get it from bone broth, though there are great plant-based options too. As I mentioned earlier, every phase of a woman's life brings new demands – and supplements, when taken with the right guidance, can be a valuable part of staying balanced and nourished.

What's most important, I've learned to seek support when I need it. Whether that means a doctor, a dermatologist, a nutritionist, or simply talking to other women going through the same thing – these conversations matter. There's no shame in prioritizing your health. In fact, there's strength in it.

Hormonal Health: Navigating the Ups and Downs

As I grow older, I've become far more conscious of my hormonal health. It's not just about mood swings or sleep issues – hormones are part of a deeply interconnected system that affects everything from metabolism to emotional well-being. One shift that's helped me navigate these changes has been incorporating intermittent fasting into my routine. I talk more about this in the chapter on food, but here's the short version: I don't do it every day, since my doctor advised against that. Practising it every other day works well for me. It helps regulate hunger and keeps me from feeling overwhelmed by constant calorie tracking.

For me, IF has helped stabilize certain hormonal patterns, especially those related to insulin and cortisol, which can fluctuate more during perimenopause. But that's my personal experience. As I've said before, wellness isn't about rigid rules. It's about tuning in to what your body needs at different stages. Some days, especially during my period or when my energy dips, I skip fasting entirely. Just like with fitness or nutrition, the key is adaptability. If you're considering IF or any new habit, consult a medical professional and take a gentle, informed approach.

Tuning in to your body's signals is key. Over the years, I've learned to notice when something feels off. When my energy dips or my mood feels heavier than usual, it often points to low vitamin D or B12 levels. I mentioned earlier how regular blood tests became part of my routine, and they've helped me stay ahead of deficiencies and feel more in control. Being proactive, especially with hormonal shifts, makes a world of difference in how you feel and function.

> For Hormonal Health: If something feels off — tiredness, irritability, sleep trouble — don't ignore it. These are often signs your body needs support. Get your levels checked and seek the right guidance. A little awareness goes a long way.

Living Full Steam Ahead After 50: Embrace the Liberation

As I step into this next phase of life, I've realized that age isn't a limitation. It's an invitation. Menopause and perimenopause don't signal the end of your vitality. If anything, they open the door to a new kind of freedom. There's wisdom in knowing who you are, in letting go of things that no longer serve you, and in embracing the possibilities still waiting ahead.

I know many women who say they're living their best lives in their fifties and beyond. I anticipate the same for myself. Whether it's exploring new places, rediscovering passions, deepening relationships, or simply living with more intention, life after 50 has its own kind of magic. As I've shared throughout this chapter, it's no longer about chasing youth. It's about owning every stage with pride, softness, and joy.

This doesn't mean everything is perfect or easy. But change, as I've experienced since my twenties, isn't something to fear. It's something to meet with awareness and grace. So to every woman wondering what lies ahead: know that the best is far from over. You're just getting started.

Final Word: A Lifelong Commitment to Health

Women's health is not a destination, it's a journey – one that continues through every phase of life. From the vibrancy of your twenties to the transformations of pregnancy, postpartum, and the wisdom that comes with menopause, it's important to honour each stage. Fitness, wellness, and self-care aren't just about how we look – they're about how we feel. Strength, flexibility, and well-being are things we can cultivate throughout our lives. Remember, it's about progress, not perfection. The key is to embrace each phase with love, patience, and respect for what our bodies are going through.

This is your life. Own it. Celebrate it. And most important, keep showing up for yourself, because a healthy, vibrant life is something you deserve at every stage of your journey.

PART III

MIND

7

Holistic Wellness: The Mind, Body, and Soul Connection

Wellness is often reduced to just physical health: how fit you are, how you look, how much you move. But real wellness is so much more than that. It's not only about the body; it's about balance – mind, body, and soul. If even one of these aspects is out of sync, everything else feels off.

For me, holistic wellness isn't about quick fixes or surface-level health trends. It's about taking care of myself in a way that supports all-round well-being – mental, emotional, and physical. Because let's be real: you can't work your way out through burnout, meditate your way out of poor nutrition, or sleep your way through chronic stress. It all has to come together.

As women, we're often expected to put everything and everyone else first, which makes it easy to neglect ourselves. But pursuing true wellness isn't selfish – it's essential. When we take care of ourselves, everything else tends to fall into place more naturally.

For me, this means nourishing movement, mindful eating, rest, stress management, and emotional well-being – all working together to help me feel my best. This chapter is all about the practices that help me stay grounded, energized, and aligned in every sense of the word. Some of them you've seen glimpses of earlier – whether in my daily rituals, skincare, or what I like to call my 'magic potions'. Here, we dive deeper into how I bring them all together to feel whole.

Rest, Boundaries, and Balance

The Guilt of Rest

I'll admit, I haven't always made my mental health a priority. Fitness and physical health were always at the top of my list, but it took me a while to realize that mental wellness needs just as much care. For years, I thrived on being constantly busy, working on new projects, travelling for shoots, juggling motherhood. I was always in motion, convinced that if I wasn't doing more, I wasn't doing enough. But eventually, I learned the hard way that rest isn't optional. It is essential.

Taking time off comes with guilt, especially for women – guilt about missing opportunities while relaxing, guilt for taking time for ourselves, guilt for not always being available for others. I used to think,

'How can I afford to rest when there's so much to do?' I'd tell myself, 'My family needs me, my work needs me.' I know many women struggle with that feeling of having to always be available. But here's the truth: you can't pour from an empty cup. If you don't take care of yourself, you're not really helping anyone.

I feel I'm professionally at my prime right now, and I'd still catch myself thinking, 'If I take time off, I'm probably missing out on something.' That mindset is exhausting and, honestly, damaging. I used to combine work with travel, thinking that if I could squeeze a vacation in between shoots, I'd be fine. But over time, I realized rest isn't about working in some leisure. It's about taking space for yourself. My friends, even my son, would remind me, 'You need to just take some time off.' And though I found it hard to stop, I finally understood the importance of listening. I'm learning to recharge, whether it's a whole weekend off or simply carving out a Sunday to reset. Now I can feel how invigorating it is. I'm tapping into another part of myself, and it feels really good.

Setting Boundaries for Mental Health

Once I understood the need for rest, the next step was creating boundaries around my time. Setting boundaries isn't selfish. It's an act of self-love. I had to learn that saying no is necessary to protect my peace. These boundaries started small: turning off my phone after 8 p.m., reading in silence, lying down and doing nothing, or making space to be alone with my family. At first, I resisted, thinking that if I didn't constantly respond to calls or messages, I would miss something important. But shutting out the noise is essential, especially in today's hyper-connected world.

Now when I feel the weight of the world pressing down, I listen to my body and allow myself to rest. If I'm mentally drained or physically tired, I don't hesitate to take a break. I've learned that doing nothing isn't laziness. It's essential for mental clarity. These small shifts are no different from the rituals I've shared earlier, whether it's to do with fitness, food, or skincare. Boundary setting is no longer a luxury. It's a non-negotiable part of my self-care.

The Art of Little Moments

Alongside setting boundaries, one of the most important lessons I've learned is that rest cannot be overlooked. I used to push through exhaustion, thinking I had to keep going, that stopping was a sign of weakness. Even when I was fatigued, I'd tell myself, 'I'm good, I'm great, I'm fine. I'll just pop in a vitamin or do some steam and I'll be OK.' But the truth is: you can't keep running on empty forever. You have to listen to your mind and body.

Rest is necessary, not just for physical recovery but also for mental clarity. Without sleep, nothing works. Your body doesn't function, your mind can't focus, and your energy crashes. When I wake up after a full night's rest, I feel invincible. In fact, it makes me better at being a mother, a professional, and a woman. Even on hectic days, if I'm tired, I'll take a power nap, whether it's between meetings or on set in my trailer. These small pauses really add up. It's not just the long breaks that matter. It's the little moments throughout the day that help me stay balanced physically, emotionally, and mentally.

Self-Care Starts with the Little Things

While rest and boundaries are crucial, self-care doesn't always require grand gestures. Often, it's the little, everyday acts that make the biggest difference: taking a walk, watching something light to unwind, or simply having a cup of tea with a friend. These small moments of joy can be deeply grounding, and they don't take much time.

Decluttering has become a quiet form of self-care for me. I feel lighter and more at peace after tidying up. It's not just about a clean space. It's about the mental clarity that comes with it. Even studies show that a clutter-free environment reduces stress and improves focus. Just a few minutes of tidying can clear your head. Journaling is another way I release stress. When I'm overwhelmed, writing things down helps me process what I'm feeling. I find it liberating. Sometimes, it's as simple as listening to music or stepping outside. Just a few minutes in nature can shift my mood completely.

I also find great peace in being outdoors. Whether it's walking in nature or simply stepping out to breathe fresh air, getting out of confined spaces resets my mind. Breathing deeply, even if the air isn't perfect, helps me feel grounded. Gardening is another simple but powerful way I reset. It allows me to connect with the earth, calm my thoughts, and find a little peace amid the chaos. And of course, there's the trusty hot shower. Always works wonders.

The Two Sides of Me: Weekdays vs Weekends

Over time, I've come to realize that I'm not the same person during the week as I am on the weekend. It's not about personality shifts, but how I manage my energy and time. From Monday to Friday, I'm in full-on work mode: focused, structured, and determined to get everything done. I thrive on routine, and having a packed schedule gives me a sense of purpose. My days are filled with meetings, shoots, and endless to-do lists, and I find satisfaction in checking tasks off one by one. By the end of the week, I've usually accomplished most of my goals, and that gives me a deep sense of fulfilment.

Weekdays: The Hustle

During the weekdays, productivity is the name of the game. I wake up early, stick to my routine, and dive into everything with purpose. Whether it's working out, taking meetings, or managing personal responsibilities, everything falls into place as planned. There's a rhythm to the weekdays that keeps me feeling aligned and on track. And because I've met my goals for the week, I also give myself permission to slow down over the weekend. That sense of accomplishment makes the rest feel well earned. The structure of the weekdays fuels me, and the discipline carries over from all the practices I've spoken about – fitness, nourishment, even skincare. But what's equally powerful is the freedom to step away from that structure.

Weekends: The Recharge

By the time the weekend arrives, I'm ready to switch gears. I allow myself the freedom to sleep in, enjoy a cheat meal, or skip the workout if I'm not feeling up to it. Weekends are my time to breathe, and I've learned that this break is essential to my well-being. The contrast between the hustle of the week and the relaxation of the weekend is what prevents me from burning out. I now consciously give myself permission to unplug. It's not that I'm doing nothing all weekend. Sometimes I'm holed up in my room, binge-watching a show, or simply taking a walk. It's about doing what feels right for me in that moment.

These small acts of rest are when I feel most relaxed and recharged. It's a chance to reset and detach from the demands of the week. I could easily get caught up in the urge to work, finish tasks, or check my email, but I now know that taking this time to recharge makes me ready for the week ahead. It's an investment in my energy and creativity, one that helps me return to Monday with a clear mind and full energy.

The Necessity of the Two Sides

I've realized that having these two distinct versions of myself isn't a flaw. It's a necessity. The weekday version of me is driven, focused, and determined to check off everything on my list. But the weekend version is just as important. Without that time to rest and reset — a theme that's come up in so many areas of wellness for me — I wouldn't be able to fully embrace the challenges of the week. These two sides work in tandem, helping me show up in my work and in my life with clarity and intention. Whether it's pushing myself during the week or allowing myself grace on the weekend, the balance is what keeps me at my best.

Guilt-Free Living for Women

As I found balance in my routine, I encountered a deeper, more complex form of guilt: the struggle of managing all my roles as a woman while maintaining my well-being. It's something so many of us can relate to. The constant pull between being a mother, partner, daughter, friend, and professional often leaves us feeling we're not doing enough. I've been there.

As we juggle multiple roles, it's easy to lose sight of ourselves. I've experienced the guilt of rushing through the day, trying to meet deadlines, care for my family, and show up for everyone — except myself. It took me years to realize that taking time for myself wasn't selfish. It was necessary. If you're not taking care of yourself, you can't give your best to anyone else. I've already said this earlier in this chapter, but it's worth repeating because we tend to forget it all too easily.

Balance, I've learned, is key. In the early years of motherhood, I felt guilty every time work took priority over my son, or when I couldn't be present for every moment. I'd rush home from shoots or meetings, hoping to make up for lost time. But what I've learned is this: it's OK to ask for help, to delegate tasks, to take breaks. Doing so doesn't make you less of a mother, partner, or professional – it makes you stronger and more present in the roles that matter most.

A huge part of maintaining my well-being has been leaning on a strong support system. My mom, my sister, my friends, even my dog – all have been my pillars, not just when things are smooth but especially during the tough times. Sometimes, all I need is someone to listen, and that alone makes all the difference. I've learned that asking for help doesn't make me weak. It makes me stronger. Their love and support give me the strength to keep going, and I've realized that I can't carry everything on my own.

The Power of Affirmations and Prayers

Tuning out the noise is key to living a balanced and peaceful life, and for me, it starts right from the first moments of the day. While much of my routine revolves around taking care of my body – whether it's health shots, breaking my fast, or simply embracing my love for mornings – there's one practice that feels truly intrinsic to who I am: my affirmations and prayers. These are not just rituals; they're a way to centre myself, reset my mind, and align my thoughts with the energy I want to carry throughout the day.

My affirmations and prayers set the tone. This practice, grounded in holistic living, aligns my energy and ensures I'm ready to tackle the challenges ahead with the right mindset. Every morning, I spend a few moments in quiet reflection, telling myself:

'I am strong, capable, and resilient.'

'I am worthy of love and success.'

'Today, I am open to new opportunities and growth.'

It's not just about saying the words, it's about internalizing them, making sure I truly believe them as I face the day. These affirmations help me recalibrate and create a positive foundation for everything I do.

But just as important as my morning affirmations is my night routine. I've always ended my day with a set of affirmations because I believe how we end the day shapes our rest and, ultimately, how we start the next. I say:

'I release the stress of the day and allow myself to rest.'

'I am grateful for the opportunities I had today, and I welcome tomorrow with open arms.'

'I am at peace with myself, and I embrace the quiet moments of rest.'

These two practices – morning and night – are powerful tools for resetting. Saying my affirmations at night provides closure to the day, while the morning affirmations offer a fresh start. They're not just routines; they're a way to stay grounded and connected to what matters most, especially when life can feel overwhelming.

Prayers hold a special place in my routine too. While affirmations set my intentions, prayers ground me and remind me of the bigger picture. I don't always follow a specific set of words, but the act of praying helps me reconnect with something greater than myself. Whether I'm asking for guidance or simply expressing gratitude, prayer brings peace in the chaos of daily life. It centres my spirit before I face the world.

In many ways, these practices – affirmations and prayers – are about setting intentions. They align my thoughts, energy, and spirit, allowing me to live holistically, with purpose, clarity, and peace. They're my compass, steering me through the noise and helping me show up as the best version of myself.

Mind, Body, Spirit: The Holistic Balance

Holistic health is about recognizing that all parts of you are connected and taking care of one part nurtures the others. For me, this approach became essential when I understood that well-being goes beyond what we see in the mirror. It's not just about eating well or working out; it's about how we feel in our minds, how we nourish our souls, and how we connect with our surroundings.

My journey into holistic living began with Ayurveda, and it truly shifted my perspective. I remember the first time I attended an Ayurveda retreat – it completely changed my understanding of wellness. Ayurveda isn't just about conventional body care. It's about understanding your unique constitution and responding to its needs with mindfulness and intention. It taught me that wellness is about nourishing every aspect of yourself, inside and out. Practices like Panchakarma, Jal Neti, and Vaman Neti help cleanse both body and mind in ways I never expected. These practices opened my eyes to the idea that wellness is an ongoing relationship with oneself.

Yoga also became transformative for me. It's not just a physical practice; it's mental and spiritual as well. Through yoga, I've learned to breathe, stay present, and truly connect with my body. Each asana, each breath, brings me back to myself, helping me process life's challenges. It reminds me to listen to my body and honour its needs. Much like my approach to fitness, this kind of movement is about tuning in, not pushing through.

Incorporating mindfulness into my daily routine has been essential in helping me live with intention. Whether it's a few quiet moments in the morning, journaling my thoughts, or simply focusing on my breath throughout the day, mindfulness keeps me grounded. It helps me appreciate the present moment and fosters a deep connection with myself. These practices aren't just checklists; they've become integral to how I approach the world.

I also cherish simple self-care rituals like herbal teas, meditation, and spending time alone. In a world that often pushes us to do more, I've learned the importance of slowing down. Whether it's enjoying a warm cup of tea, taking a mindful walk (a small ritual I spoke about in the 'Magic Potions' chapter), or breathing deeply for a few minutes, these moments help me stay balanced.

Discipline and Consistency: The Building Blocks of Success

People often ask me how I manage to keep going, year after year. They look at me and wonder, 'Don't you ever feel tired? Or just want to take a break?' And every time, I smile and think to myself, 'If only they knew my secret.'

So here it is – the secret that fuels me, even on the toughest days. It's discipline and consistency.

Yes, I've said it before and I'll say it again – because it's that important. Whether we're talking about food, fitness, beauty, or wellness, consistency is the common thread. It's not just one of the tools in the box. It is the foundation. Without it, nothing else holds.

Discipline, for me, is the art of creating structure in my life. It's about establishing habits and routines that align with my long-term goals. It's the force that gets me to rise early for my workout, to make healthy choices, and to stay focused on what matters. Consistency is the commitment to show up every single day. It's about doing the things that support my well-being, even when the results aren't immediately visible.

I often recall what Terence Lewis once shared about me on *Moving in with Malaika*. He spoke about how, even 25 years ago, I'd always be the first one at dance class – even before him. It wasn't just about showing up. It was about being there with discipline and passion, every single day. He said that punctuality, that commitment to being prepared always, set me apart. I carry that discipline and commitment with me in everything I do. For me, it's not about being perfect. It's about being persistent, no matter how things feel in the moment.

Discipline and consistency have taught me patience. I thrive on structure. Whether it's my workout routine, my meals, or my mental well-being, sticking to what I've set for myself helps me stay on track. It's a way of showing up for myself. And even on days when I fall short, I know the next day is a new opportunity to try again.

Learning to Validate Your Own Worth

It's not all smooth sailing though. There are times when I find myself questioning everything, feeling down or discouraged. There are days where I just don't want to do anything. I don't want to see anybody's face. I feel upset or out of shape. I feel low, sad, or just generally horrible.

But I've learned to pull myself out of it. I tell myself that maybe, just maybe, I have it better than someone else. And even though that doesn't erase what I'm feeling, it helps me shift perspective. Just because I may have it better doesn't mean my struggles aren't valid. We all have our own battles. But I remind myself that I have so many opportunities in life, and I'm not going to waste any of them.

I remind myself every time that consistency is the glue that holds everything together. I tell myself, 'If I don't want to waste this opportunity, the only way not to waste it is by waking up, showing up, and bringing my best self forward.' That's the only way I won't waste the day, and I'll avoid letting an opportunity slip away.

It's at those times that I remind myself to 'slap' the motivation into myself, quite literally. I joke about getting someone to slap me two or three times to get going, but honestly, sometimes that's how you have to treat yourself – like your own biggest cheerleader. You can't wait for someone else to validate your efforts. You've got to validate yourself.

Once again, it's not about doing everything perfectly. It's about showing up. And that's the most important part. Whether it's a workout, a meal, or a mental reset, consistency is what keeps me on track. Even if I'm not seeing the progress I want, I keep going. Because the truth is, some days will be harder than others. That's the reality of life, and it's OK.

Rewriting the Narrative on Body Image

As much as I talk about consistency and discipline, there's something else that often lurks in the background – comparison. We live in a world that constantly pressures us to meet certain beauty standards, and it's something I had to learn to navigate in my own journey.

Social media, the public eye, and society as a whole put so much pressure on us to look a certain way. It's easy to get caught up in the numbers on the scale or in the unrealistic portrayals of 'perfection' that we see. But over time, I've recognized that it's not about looking a certain way. It's about feeling strong, confident, and healthy in my own body – something I touched on in both my fitness and hormonal health journeys.

I've had my struggles with body image, just like so many women. I've had days where I look in the mirror and feel less than great about what I see. But I've realized that our worth isn't determined by the way we look. It's about how we feel in our skin and how we carry ourselves with confidence, regardless of size or shape.

We've all been there, right? You feel you're doing everything right – working out, eating healthy, taking care of your mind – but the mirror doesn't show what you expect. The weight isn't coming off, your body doesn't feel different, and you can't help but ask yourself, 'Why isn't this working?'

That's when the frustration sets in. But I've learned something important: there's no quick fix.

It's all about showing up, doing your best, and trusting the process. We live in a world of instant gratification, where results are expected right away. But true transformation takes time.

When my friends share their struggles with body image, I always tell them this: if you're doing everything right, working hard, staying consistent, and still not seeing the results, it may be time to take a deeper look. Sometimes there's a medical issue that's preventing change. I always recommend checking in with a healthcare professional — as I did during my own health journey.

But beyond that, I remind them that the journey is not a sprint — it's a marathon. This is why consistency is so important. On the days you feel like giving up because you don't see it going anywhere, that's when you need to remind yourself why you started in the first place.

You have to be your own biggest cheerleader. I've stopped relying on external validation. We all need to find that inner strength, that voice that says, 'I love myself, I'm doing my best, and I'm worthy of all the good things coming my way.' You need to have a love affair with yourself! That's the kind of affirmation that pushes you forward, even when the road gets tough.

> So my advice? Stop comparing. Stop waiting for someone else to validate your efforts. It's OK not to see the results immediately, but don't stop. Keep showing up, and trust that consistency will get you there. It is most important to love yourself through the journey, even when things aren't perfect. That's where the true transformation lies.

Routine: Your Guide to Consistency

Building the mental and emotional foundation for well-being was just the start. What keeps everything aligned and moving forward is the structure I create in my daily life. Routine is the framework I depend on to stay grounded and purposeful, especially when life feels chaotic. I thrive on routine. Having a set schedule gives me a sense of purpose. It gives me a reason to wake up each day and know that I'm working towards something. But that doesn't mean I'm inflexible. It's about finding a system that works for me, while leaving room for life to happen.

Routine has always been a part of my life, but I've learned that the key to staying productive, healthy, and aligned is not seeing it as a restriction. It's a supportive system that holds everything else together – just like consistency, which I've spoken about so often throughout this book. Whether it's waking up at a certain time, having my meals at set intervals, or practising yoga regularly, this structure ensures that I stay on track with my health and personal goals. Some might think it's too rigid, but for me, it's a practice that allows me to be my best self.

That said, flexibility is also crucial. I've come to understand that it's OK to deviate from the routine once in a while – whether it's taking a nap or treating myself to something indulgent. Life is all about balance. Flexibility within structure helps me stay grounded and not overwhelmed. It's not about rigid perfection. It's about creating a framework that works and adjusting when needed.

A Work in Progress

With every lesson, challenge, and success, I've come to realize that I'm not looking for perfection. The beauty of this journey lies in being a work in progress – a constant evolution towards becoming a better version of myself. I'm always evolving, always learning, and embracing that journey. I may not have all the answers, and I may not always get it right, but I'm constantly striving to be better. Every day is an opportunity to grow, improve, and become the best version of myself.

As I look back on my life, there are things I wish I had continued pursuing – like hobbies or activities I once loved but eventually let go of. Whether it was my love for track and field, dance, or pottery, life and other priorities took over. I now understand that I could've balanced those hobbies with my career and other responsibilities. I regret not sticking with them longer.

But I also know that every decision I've made has shaped the person I am today. Those things I let go of were part of the process, and while they don't define me, they contributed to my growth. I've realized that it's important to honour the choices I make, even if they're not always perfect, and embrace what I've gained from each step of the journey.

So my advice to anyone reading this is simple: don't be too hard on yourself. Embrace the process. We're all works in progress, and that's the beauty of it. You don't have to have it all figured out right away. You just have to keep going.

Final Word

I want to leave you with one final thought: wellness is a lifelong journey, not a destination. It takes patience, compassion, and a deep connection between mind, body, and soul. True wellness isn't just about appearance or fitness – it's about balance, nurturing your mental well-being, and learning to slow down. Rest is essential for your health, and mental health is just as important as physical health. Prioritizing it helps you stay steady and present through life's many seasons.

There will be ups and downs, and that's OK. Progress doesn't always look dramatic – it's often made in quiet, consistent moments. Every small step you take brings you closer to the version of yourself you're meant to grow into.

So listen to your body. Give yourself the grace to pause and replenish. Honour your mental and emotional well-being. Trust the rhythm of your life and embrace the journey with kindness. Growth takes time. You've got this!

8
Unapologetically Me: My Life, Unfiltered

In life, no matter how many accolades you've earned or how disciplined your routine, it's the people you love and trust who truly anchor you. For me, those anchors have always been my family and friends – my mom, my sister, and my closest circle – who offer love, stability, and unwavering support. In a world full of noise, these relationships keep me grounded. They remind me of who I am, especially in moments when I lose sight of it. They are my therapy, helping me reset when life feels overwhelming.

Having people who listen, who truly listen, is a rare blessing. There's immense power in knowing someone has your back. They don't necessarily have to offer solutions. Sometimes all you need is to hear, 'You're not alone in this.' These relationships are a constant reminder that no matter how crazy life gets, I have a safe space to simply be myself. And this, I believe, is integral to mental well-being: having a strong, supportive network to help preserve clarity, especially when the world feels chaotic.

The People Who Raise Me Up

I've never been someone who opens up easily. Vulnerability was never a trait I wore proudly. As a 'true-blue Scorpio', I've always kept things close to my chest, processing emotions on my own, in my own time. But over the years, I've learned that sharing my thoughts, feelings, and moments of uncertainty with the people closest to me isn't a weakness – it's been one of the most liberating experiences of my life. There's no shame in feeling low or unsure, and I've had my fair share of self-doubt. But one thing has remained constant: the unwavering support of those I love.

Above all, my son, Arhaan, is my emotional anchor. He is my heart, my grounding force. Being his mother has taught me more than I could ever have imagined – patience, unconditional love, and an entirely new perspective on life. Arhaan has given me a lens through which I see the world differently, from the simple joy of hearing him laugh to the profound moments when he shares his thoughts with me. He's growing up fast, but the quiet, simple moments we share – watching movies or chatting about his day – are what truly matter. No matter how busy life gets or how much the world changes, he will always be my constant.

Our bond has been my strength through life's changes. When I went through my divorce, I was deeply concerned about how it would affect him. What I didn't expect was how much he'd grow from it – how understanding and resilient he's been. Even as a child, he spent a lot of time with my mom, Joyce, whose home became his sanctuary. Arhaan has always had this incredible ability to see the good in everything. He's the one who reminds me of what truly matters in life: loving unconditionally and being present for the people who matter most.

I'll never forget a moment before my stand-up comedy set. I was incredibly nervous, consumed by the fear of failure. I kept thinking, 'Something bad is going to happen. I'm going to embarrass myself.' I called Arhaan, but he didn't pick up. All I wanted was to hear his calming voice. When he finally called back, his words were exactly what I needed: 'You've got this, Mom!' Just hearing that was enough for me to shake off my nerves and step onto the stage with confidence. It's moments like these that remind me how important it is to have someone who believes in you, especially when you're filled with doubt. Arhaan is wise beyond his years.

Then there's my sister, Amrita. She is one of the strongest pillars in my life – personally and professionally. We've been through everything together, from childhood squabbles to supporting each other through life's toughest moments. Whether offering advice, sharing a laugh, or simply being there in silence, Amrita has always been a source of comfort. What makes our bond so special isn't just words – it's presence. We've shared so many precious moments: tears, laughter, joy, frustration. Through it all, we've always found comfort in each other. She's not just my sister – she's my best friend and my confidante.

Arhaan and Amrita share a bond that's like no other. They're not just aunt and nephew – they're best friends. Arhaan confides in her about things he doesn't want to share with me, and I love the understanding and friendship they have. There's a natural ease between them, and they support each other in ways only close-knit family can. I'm so grateful for the role Ammu plays in his life. She's like a second mother to him, and it warms my heart to see their connection.

Arhaan doesn't bottle things up. If something is weighing on him, he'll let me know sooner or later. He's open, chill, and honest, and I'm so thankful for that kind of communication. I always remind him that no matter what happens, I'll always be here for him. He knows he can share anything with me.

Then there's my mother, Joyce. She's been my rock from day one. I can't even express how much her love and support have meant to me. She was there when I had Arhaan, offering emotional strength and practical help. I remember those early days of motherhood when I was trying to balance work and being a new mom – she stepped in without hesitation. She helped raise Arhaan with a sense of calm and care that only she could offer. Her wisdom, her presence, and her unwavering love have been a source of strength for Arhaan and me. The most important lesson my mom taught me was the power of choice. She raised us to respect others but also to never be afraid to speak our minds, live life on our terms, and make decisions with confidence. That's something I've carried with me through every chapter of my life. As a family, we've shared so many memories – celebrations, loss, love, laughter. Of course, we've had our disagreements, but at the end of the day, our bond is unshakeable. I know that no matter what, they will always have my back.

Beyond my family, I've been lucky to have strong friendships within the industry. Kareena Kapoor, Karisma Kapoor, Dino Morea, and Neha Dhupia have been integral to my journey. These are friends who've seen me at my best and my lowest – and never judged. They've lent me their ears, offered shoulders to cry on, and given me something to laugh about when I needed it most. These bonds go far beyond the superficial. They're built on years of shared experiences, mutual respect, and unconditional love. Kareena and Karisma, in particular, have stood by me through some of my most difficult phases. Whether helping me navigate the pressures of the public eye or just showing up for a girls' night to recharge, their support has meant the world to me. Neha too has played a huge role – always reminding me to take care of myself, to love myself a little harder. We've all had our ups and downs, but our friendship is grounded in loyalty and care.

I also have friends outside the industry who've been just as essential to my joy – Vikram Phadnis, Aditi Govitrikar, Delnaz Daruwala, Vinaj Bijlani, and Anuja Bijlani. We meet often to laugh, play games, and just be ourselves. This is my crazy, happy place – where I can be vulnerable, goofy, and free, without any need for pretence.

Seema Sajdeh, my former sister-in-law, continues to hold a special place in my life. Despite our family ties shifting, she remains family to me. Seema has always been forthright, direct, and sincere – traits I deeply admire. Our relationship has grown with time, built on shared memories, mutual support, and an evolving sense of respect. Arhaan shares a beautiful bond with Seema, just like he does with Ammu. They connect through humour and affection, and it brings me joy to see them laughing and being themselves around each other. It reminds me that family doesn't have to follow rigid definitions – what matters is love, connection, and presence.

And finally, there's Casper, my dog. He's been by my side for over 10 years, and I truly can't imagine life without him. His quiet companionship has been a steady comfort through every high and low. It was Arhaan who wanted a dog, and though I was hesitant at first, I'm so glad we welcomed Casper into our home. He reminds me of how beautiful and grounding the simplest joys in life can be.

Moving On with Grace: Life After Divorce

Yes, I had a very public divorce – and yes, it wasn't easy. The decision to divorce Arbaaz wasn't easy either, but after much reflection, it became clear that it was the best choice for me, for him, and for our son. It wasn't about failure. It was about recognizing that sometimes relationships reach a point where they no longer contribute to anyone's growth or happiness. We shared a history, a child, and memories that will forever bind us, but love alone wasn't enough to keep us together.

What proved most challenging was not the decision itself, but the toll it took privately and publicly. I kept the separation to myself for a while, fearing the judgement that would come. But when the rumours grew louder, I could no longer stay silent. Speaking up was like lifting a weight, but the damage in terms of how people viewed me had already been done.

Divorce, especially under public scrutiny, comes with its own set of challenges: the judgement, the invasive headlines, and the trolling. But the most difficult part wasn't the media frenzy. It was the pressure of constantly being watched, analysed, and criticized for making a deeply personal decision. It was painful to be dragged through the mud for something that should have remained private.

What mattered most was how I handled the situation. The decision to separate was made with love and respect for Arbaaz. We both knew that our happiness needed to come first, not just for us, but for our son. Arhaan was always our priority. Explaining the divorce to him was the hardest part. No child should have to experience that, but I made sure he felt loved, safe, and secure during such a turbulent time. No matter what, his home would always be full of love.

Co-parenting with Arbaaz is something I'm proud of. Though we aren't best friends, we've built a healthy and respectful relationship for Arhaan's sake. Our bond is rooted in mutual respect. Arbaaz is still very much a part of my family. He shares a special bond with my mom, and my family still consider him family. That kind of respect is what has allowed us to navigate this chapter of our lives.

The separation was emotionally taxing, but it was also liberating. It forced me to open up, not just to those around me, but to myself. I learned that vulnerability doesn't make you weak. It makes you human. Sharing my emotions with my loved ones became one of the most healing aspects of this journey.

The best advice I received during this time came from my family and close friends. They never questioned my decision to leave. They simply said, 'You're strong. You're making the right choice for you.' But the worst advice came from those who projected their doubts onto me. They asked, 'Are you sure about this?' And while their concerns weren't malicious, they made the process harder than it needed to be. At the end of the day, it was my decision, and I had to trust that it was the right one.

The years after the divorce taught me a lot about self-worth. I no longer felt the need to rush into a relationship to validate myself. I focused on rediscovering who I was, on what made me happy. I wasn't in search of Mr Right but of becoming 'right' for myself. I wanted to grow, to find my own path, and to learn about myself without the pressure of being in a relationship.

To all the women out there, especially those who are newly divorced, here's my message: don't wait for someone to complete you. You're already whole. Society places immense pressure on women to be in a relationship, but it's OK to live life on your own terms. You don't need a partner to define your worth.

Ending a relationship is not the end of the world. It's an opportunity for a new beginning. I'm proud of how far I've come, and I know I'm a better person because of it. My journey post-divorce has taught me strength, resilience, and the importance of taking care of myself so I can be there for those I love. I am not defined by my divorce. I'm defined by how I choose to live my life moving forward.

On Arjun Kapoor

Life has a way of taking you down unexpected paths, and sometimes those paths lead to people who teach you lessons you didn't even know you needed. Arjun Kapoor was one of those people. Our relationship was a significant, meaningful chapter in my life. We were open about our relationship, and it felt natural at the time to share parts of our journey with the world. We talked about our future, even about marriage, but life has a way of unfolding differently than expected. Sometimes, things change, and it's OK to accept that.

What's important to me is that our relationship was built on love and respect. Arjun became close with my family – my son, my sister, my friends – and I've always appreciated the bond he shared with them. I hold dear and will always value the connection he had with my loved ones. Just because something ends doesn't mean there's bitterness or animosity. Like many things, relationships can run their course. That's life.

We've both moved on, and I've learned that while vulnerability is important, there are parts of life we prefer to keep private. We don't owe anyone answers, and the way we choose to navigate our personal lives is our choice. What matters is the love and respect we still have for each other, and that's all I'm willing to say at this point. At the end of the day, it's about growth, understanding, and moving forward with dignity. I've found my peace, and I hope he has too.

The Price of Public Life

Living in the public eye means your life is constantly under a microscope, and let me tell you, that is exhausting. Early in my career, I was labelled 'sexy'.

Fine, I embraced it. Over time, I realized how the term 'item number' became synonymous with objectification. We're more than just the labels society has put on us.

The end of my marriage to Arbaaz marked the beginning of a nasty and relentless media frenzy. The gossip, judgement, and insensitive headlines took their toll. The hardest part wasn't the speculation – it was the overwhelming, suffocating feeling of being constantly watched and analysed by the world. For months after the divorce, I chose silence, hoping the dust would settle. But in return, I faced harsh, unforgiving judgement from people who had no idea what I was truly going through. I was criticized for making a personal decision that was mine alone. The pressure of living under such scrutiny was unbearable at times. Women often face this harsh, invasive judgement – personal, probing, and, frankly, lacking any understanding. I wasn't immune to that.

The most important lesson I've learned: block out the noise. But let me be clear, it's not easy to ignore the noise. Not by a long shot. The world never stops talking, never stops judging, and it can be overwhelming. But you learn. You have to. I surrounded myself with the right people – my mom, my sister, my son, close friends, and even my dog.

They became my sanctuary. They help me stay grounded, and they remind me of what truly matters: my happiness, my peace of mind, and my health. With their unwavering support, I found my peace, my strength. They keep me focused on what's important – not the trolls, not the haters. I stopped trying to meet societal expectations or please people who have no place in my life. The decisions I make, how I live, and how I present myself are MY choices, and I refuse to apologize for them.

The judgement doesn't stop there. People will always find something to criticize – whether it's my relationships, my choices, or even something as ridiculous as my 'duck walk'. It's like an endless, unwelcome invasion of privacy. But guess what? I don't let it bother me any more. I've learned how to block out the negativity, to focus on what truly matters, and to protect myself with the love and support of those who truly understand me. My mantra is simple: 'No guts, no glory.' People will comment, say what they want, but at the end of the day, their opinions don't define me. They never will.

And the taunts? I've been mocked for everything. My complexion, my body, my choices – none of it is off-limits. Growing up, I was often teased because I was slightly darker in complexion than my younger sister, Amrita. *'Arre aapki beti itni sawali hai. Aise kaise? Ammu toh kitni gori hai!'* I've heard it all. These judgements are part of the territory, and I no longer waste energy on them. What matters is the love I receive from my family and friends. They've got my back, and theirs are the only opinions I care about.

Let's talk about the internet too. Social media has created a toxic environment. The anonymity of these platforms lets trolls hide behind screens and hurl insults. While I've learned to ignore the negativity, not everyone can handle it. Cyberbullying is a serious issue, especially for younger generations. It's an attack on their self-esteem and identity. And let me tell you, as a mother, when someone comes for my kid, my fangs come out. I don't take that lightly. I am thick-skinned, but trolls don't realize the lasting damage they can do, especially to young minds. When people target my son, Arhaan, for no reason, I won't stand for it. That's where I draw the line. No one has the right to mess with my family.

I've spent enough time letting people's judgements define me. No more. It's time we all stop letting society's narrow expectations control our lives. Whether it's our appearance, relationships, or how we live – we should never let judgement decide our worth. It's about self-respect, self-empowerment. And it's about standing up for who we are, no matter what the world may think.

Rewriting the Rules of Relevance

One thing I'll never understand is society's obsession with a woman's age. Why is it such a big deal? Why should I be judged for living life on my own terms? I wear what makes me happy, continue working because it fulfils me, and live my life the way I choose. But for some reason, society feels the need to scrutinize women in their forties and fifties for doing the same things that younger women or men of all ages get a free pass for.

The judgement women face is not only about age. It's especially harsh when it comes to major life events. When a woman chooses to pursue something new – whether it's a fresh relationship, a career change, or simply a new passion – society is quick to judge, question, or even criticize. 'How could she?' is what most ask in disbelief. A man, on the other hand, is lauded for his 'second act', but a woman is often met with scepticism. This double standard is something I've come to recognize and reject.

Here's the truth: I don't care any more. For long, I tried to make others comfortable with my decisions.

But now I do what's right for me and the people I love. I've learned not to apologize for living authentically. I'm done trying to meet anyone's standards or conform to outdated norms. Society's obsession with age and appearance doesn't define me. And I won't let it.

We're often pressured to remain 'relevant', to fit into someone else's version of who we should be. But relevance isn't about looking younger or ticking the right boxes. It's about staying true to yourself, evolving, and embracing who you are at any stage of life. Confidence isn't about perfection. It's about owning your story and letting your authenticity shine.

I've also faced judgements that go beyond age and choices. People have labelled me with terms like 'bechari' (poor thing), but that's not how I roll. I've risen above my challenges, just like every woman does. I'm not asking for sympathy. I'm asking for respect. I refuse to conform to stereotypes about how women should look, act, or live their lives. We've been conditioned from a young age to fit into prescribed moulds, but it's time we break free from those expectations.

I feel more confident, empowered, and alive now than I ever have. I'm embracing who I am – my age, my choices, my look – and doing it unapologetically.

I feel more comfortable in my skin than ever before, and I'm owning it. I've chosen to let go of society's obsession with youth and the way it impacts women's self-worth. Ageing doesn't diminish a woman's value. It amplifies her strength and wisdom. Age is just a number, and I've proven time and again that I'm not defined by it or by my appearance. I feel good in my skin, and that's all that matters.

To every woman out there: don't wait for someone to define your worth. Live life on your terms, embrace your true self, and be proud of the woman you've become. Age, relationships, career choices – they don't define you. What defines you is your strength, your authenticity, and your refusal to conform. Let go of those old rules, embrace your unique journey, and live unapologetically. You are enough, just as you are.

Healing Through Connection

Following my divorce in May 2017, I embarked on a journey of self-discovery and healing, a process that deepened during the global COVID-19 pandemic. For the first time, I was truly alone, holed up by myself – something I typically enjoy every now and then. But this was different. The pandemic made it clear that isolation was not as pleasant as it usually is, and it hit harder than I expected, just as it did for millions of others.

During this time, I witnessed many women grappling with mental health challenges ranging from anxiety to depression, and I saw how important it was to talk openly about mental well-being. It was a time of collective hardship, but it also gave me a chance to reflect and grow. I found myself engaging deeply in conversations that made me realize how vital it is to share our struggles. Through Sarva Yoga, a platform dedicated to promoting mental health awareness, I was able to participate in programmes that not only impacted others but helped me in the process as well.

Connecting with so many women who were open about their struggles allowed me to see just how much healing begins with talking about it. Women tend to be more emotionally sensitive and empathetic, and I felt a real connection with those who shared their stories. But I also noticed a significant gap: many men were less willing to talk about their mental health, likely because they perceive it as a weakness. I believe this divide needs to change, and I'm proud that Sarva Yoga has created a safe space to engage in these vital conversations.

The more I connected with others, the more I realized how much healing comes from expressing ourselves. Sharing experiences and listening to others helps break down isolation and shame. It's how we begin to heal – together. That's why I'm so proud of what we've built at Sarva Yoga, where we've contributed to the conversation about mental health and have offered support to those who need it most.

At first, when friends frequently checked in on me, I found it tedious and, honestly, a bit irritating. I felt fine and didn't think I needed constant checking in, especially when I believed I was holding up just fine. But as time passed, especially during the emotional turmoil of my divorce, I began to realize how important these check-ins were. It wasn't just about the questions – they gave me space to express myself without judgement and reminded me that someone cared enough to ask how I was really doing. I learned that emotional support isn't a sign of weakness; it's a necessity. These moments taught me to value my support system even more. It was through these conversations that I began to truly appreciate the importance of leaning on others when I needed help.

I've always been fortunate to have a strong support system – my family, my closest friends, and my son. These people have been my anchors, especially when it seemed the world was watching and judging. My close-knit circle of friends – my 'girl gang', as I call them — has been there for me during tough times, offering emotional comfort and a chance to laugh, cry, and share moments without any filter. These friendships have been a constant source of solace, reminding me that I'm not alone, even when I feel isolated in the public eye.

These deep friendships and familial bonds have allowed me to navigate the complexities of being a mother and dealing with public scrutiny. Whether it's advice or a listening ear to vent to, they've been there for me without hesitation. They know me better than I know myself, and I truly believe they've played a key role in my emotional well-being. They've always been my safe space, reminding me of the importance of connecting with others during times of hardship.

While the support from my family and friends has been essential in helping me through tough times, I've also realized that healing isn't only about receiving support — it's about opening up, being vulnerable, and allowing myself to lean into that vulnerability. And it's in those moments that I've found the most growth. The importance of embracing my emotions wasn't something I fully understood until I went through some of the most challenging times of my life. Vulnerability, I've learned, isn't a sign of weakness — it's a powerful act that has allowed me to truly heal.

Coping with Life's Curveballs

When life hits you with unexpected emotional and mental challenges, it can feel overwhelming. During moments of intense public scrutiny, emotional upheaval, and personal loss – especially during my divorce – I faced some of my toughest emotional lows. The pressure of living under a constant microscope, where every decision was open to judgement, took a significant toll.

In those moments, anxiety and stress crept in. The weight of it all often felt unbearable. There were days when the relentless criticism would drag me down, and I had to maintain composure even when I felt broken inside. The media circus and constant public judgement made it harder to process my emotions, and I realized I couldn't carry that weight alone.

It's at times like these that my holistic practices come to my rescue. The mindfulness, affirmations, and yoga I've integrated into my life have been my grounding forces. They helped me navigate those emotional storms, offering clarity, peace, and a way to release tension. These practices are my toolkit for dealing with life's curveballs. They allow me to stay connected to my inner strength and find balance, even when the world feels unbalanced.

Yoga became my sanctuary during these emotionally tumultuous times. It wasn't just about the postures – it was about grounding myself, clearing my mind, and finding peace amid the chaos. Yoga gave me space to release stress and connect with myself, offering a way to process the emotional weight without judgement. Through breath work, meditation, and movement, yoga helped me manage anxiety, stress, and self-doubt. It didn't solve everything overnight, but it helped me take steady steps towards emotional healing.

Along with yoga, taking time for myself became equally important. I realized that I needed solitude to recharge – whether it was through quiet reflection or simply by being alone with my thoughts. Taking this time allowed me to sit with my emotions and gain clarity. While it wasn't always easy to open up right away, this solitude gave me the perspective I needed to understand my struggles better.

What This Journey Taught Me

You know, sometimes life gives you lemons, and you're left scrambling to figure out how to deal with the emotional chaos. But through it all, one thing became crystal clear: it's OK not to have everything figured out. We all have our moments, and that's perfectly fine. I had to learn that I don't always need to be 'on' or have it all together – and that's where a lot of my growth happened.

What I found was strength, not the kind that comes from putting on a brave face all the time but the kind that comes from allowing myself to be vulnerable. That was a game changer. I learned to embrace my emotional strength, and in doing so, I found healing in places I never thought to look. It wasn't about having all the answers; it was about giving myself the space to heal without rushing it.

Self-care is more than bubble baths and good meals. It's about recognizing when I'm struggling and allowing myself to feel those emotions. That's when the real healing begins. By connecting with the people who truly care about me, reflecting on my own journey, and making time for practices like yoga and quiet introspection – things I've talked about before – I was able to rebuild my inner peace. It wasn't immediate, and it wasn't easy, but every step felt like a small victory.

I've learned that emotional healing isn't linear. It's messy and unpredictable, and that's OK. It's about going at your own pace, being kind to yourself, and understanding that it's a process, not a destination. Life doesn't pause for you to heal. You have to carve out that space in the middle of the chaos.

This journey also helped me grow as a person. I became more in touch with myself – my triggers, my emotions, and the moments when I needed to lean on others. As someone who tends to process things internally, I learned that opening up doesn't make you weak; it makes you stronger. It's about saying, 'I'm not alone in this,' and that, in itself, is incredibly empowering.

While I've leaned on others, I also made time for self-reflection. Those quiet moments were just as essential. They gave me clarity to process my emotions in a way that felt right for me. And honestly, a good crying session works wonders for mental clarity. I stopped bottling things up because I realized that letting my emotions out was part of the healing process. No shame in that. A good cry truly works wonders.

Through it all, I've learned that emotional well-being isn't about pushing through or pretending to be OK. It's about understanding yourself better and giving yourself permission to heal, in your own time and your own way. I used to think I had to handle everything on my own. But over time, I realized that leaning on people I trust is one of the best things I can do for myself. It's not about doing it all solo.

This journey also taught me how I want to show up for others. It's one thing to receive support, but I've learned the importance of giving it too. I try to be there for my loved ones, offering them the same safe, non-judgemental space they gave me. Through that, I've come to understand how powerful human connection can be in the healing process. Sometimes, just listening to someone's story is enough to remind you that you're not alone.

Finally, the most important lesson: you are enough. Whether you're in a relationship or not, whether you're 25 or 50, you are whole and complete. No one else can define your worth. I used to feel that I had to live up to society's expectations – but now I know that true fulfilment comes from within. We are all constantly evolving, and that's what makes us strong.

This is the message I want to share: live life on your terms, be unapologetically yourself, and find strength in your own vulnerability. Life is messy, and it's not always easy – but how we choose to move forward is what defines us. And the more we lean into that truth, the more we heal, grow, and thrive.

Final Word

At the heart of it all, the relationships that support us – our family, friends, and loved ones – are what keep us grounded and help us grow through life's challenges. These connections are built on love, respect, and understanding, offering us strength, healing, and the freedom to live authentically. Through vulnerability and mutual support, we learn that no matter what changes or hurdles we face, we are never alone. The key is to embrace those who uplift us and to always remember that real power lies in meaningful connections.

Conclusion

I've always said this: feeling good isn't a luxury. It's the most basic form of self-respect. And yet, so many of us are taught to treat wellness as an indulgence, time-consuming, or out of reach. We associate it with extremes: gruelling workouts, flawless skin, rigid diets, or spiritual enlightenment. But the truth is far simpler. Feeling good is about creating space in your life for what helps you feel strong, clear, balanced, and calm. That's it. That's the goal.

This book has been my way of opening up the doors to everything that has helped me along the way. The rituals that anchor me, the foods that fuel me, the practices that reset me, the mindset shifts that remind me who I am — each chapter has been a window into my world but more important an invitation into your own. Because this isn't a manual or a plan to follow. It's a framework to reflect, adapt, and evolve with.

When I look back at everything we've covered, a few patterns stand out. Not because I planned them that way, but because they naturally kept surfacing, and maybe that's the point. What works for us tends to repeat. We return to the same habits, the same reminders, the same truths, in different ways, at different times. And what you've probably noticed by now is that wellness isn't separate from your life. It is your life: woven into your mornings, your meals, your movement, your mindset.

We talked about beauty, yes, but not the surface-level kind. We talked about rituals. About listening to your skin, not punishing it. About treating your face and body as extensions of how you feel inside. From scrubs and shots to oils and ubtans, none of it was about changing who you are. It was about showing up for yourself with care.

We explored food and fitness, but not through the lens of control. Instead, we looked at nourishment: how to move from a place of joy, how to eat to feel alive, not ashamed. We talked about strength, about balance, about honouring what your body needs today, not punishing it for what it can't do yet.

And we spent time with the mind, with silence, stillness, softness. We talked about boundaries, about saying no, about acknowledging fatigue and heartbreak and rage and joy and letting it all belong. We made space for grief and healing. For growth and reinvention. For second chances.

As I've said before, wellness doesn't ask for perfection. It asks for presence. That you show up, even imperfectly. That you listen, even when it's inconvenient. That you pause, even when the world is rushing past. That you care enough to try.

I know it's a lot. Maybe you've underlined things. Maybe you've bookmarked a few rituals. Maybe you've read through it all and thought, 'OK ... but now what?'

That's a very real feeling.

Because often, when we consume a lot of knowledge or inspiration, there's a moment of pause at the end – a hesitation. Where do I start? What if I get it wrong? What if I can't keep it up?

If you're there right now, this is for you.

Let's Bridge the Gap: From Knowing to Doing

You don't have to overhaul your life. You don't need a 12-week plan or a new wardrobe or the perfect journal. You just need to start with one or two small, intentional steps – the kind that feel doable, repeatable, and true to you. Here are a few places you could begin:

1. Plan your meals when you're calm, not when you're starving. It sounds simple, but this is a game changer. Keep two to three go-to meals in your back pocket: meals you enjoy and can make with minimal prep. Don't wait

until you're hangry and overwhelmed. Make a loose meal outline on Sunday. Keep soaked nuts and a few washed veggies handy. Freeze that broth. Batch-roast some sweet potatoes. A little prep makes choosing better meals easier.
2. **Drink a glass of water before you eat or shop.** Not to curb appetite, but to tune into what your body really needs. Thirst often disguises itself as hunger or cravings. The next time you reach for a salty snack or start loading your cart with extras, ask: 'Have I had water today?'
3. **Get in your steps – but do it your way.** Maybe you're not clocking 10,000 steps a day, and that's OK. Can you take the stairs instead of the lift once today? Walk while you're on a phone call? Dance while brushing your teeth? Movement doesn't have to be a workout. It just has to happen.
4. **Prioritize natural light and real rest.** Open your windows when you wake up. Step outside for five minutes without your phone. Sunlight anchors your circadian rhythm. It affects your energy, mood, hormones, and sleep. Just five minutes can shift your entire day. And at night? Try dimming lights an hour before bed. Trade scrolling for stretching. Put your phone on the other side of the room.

5. Look at food before you look at supplements. You don't need to buy every trending capsule or powder. Start with whole foods. Eat more fibre. Add a spoon of soaked chia or flax to your meals. Bring in healthy fats. Ask yourself if you're eating foods that support your skin, hair, gut, and energy, and build from there.
6. Filter the noise. Not every post on the internet is the gospel. And not every influencer knows what works for you. Be curious, not compliant. Before you try something new, ask: 'Does this align with how I want to feel?' Trust your gut more than your feed.
7. Return with grace, not guilt. Did you skip your workout? Eat out three nights in a row? Forget to meditate for a week? That doesn't erase all the good you've done. It doesn't make you lazy or undisciplined. It makes you human. The goal isn't to be perfect – it's to return to yourself with more grace than guilt, again and again.

None of these are revolutionary. And they don't need to be. The point isn't to change your life overnight. The point is to keep returning to yourself – patiently, consistently, gently.

That's what I've done, time and again. Through career highs and heartbreaks, through postpartum and public scrutiny, through accidents and reinventions and everything in between, I've just kept showing up. Some days were messy. Some were beautiful. Most were a mix of both. But I've learned to trust the process. And more important, to trust myself.

And that's what I want for you. To feel at home in your skin. To feel strong in your body. To feel clear in your mind. And to know, deep down, that you are not broken, not behind, and definitely not alone.

Like I said earlier: you are enough. And you're not alone. That truth bears repeating.

So start small. Stay kind. Keep going.

And remember, it really is easy to be healthy. You just have to begin.

About the Author

In a world increasingly driven by curated perfection and manufactured narratives, the very idea of a woman walking through life with genuine, untamed grace feels almost revolutionary. And this is exactly how Malaika Arora moves through the world.

For decades, she has been a defining figure in the Indian media landscape, a presence whose infectious energy and unfazed charm command every room she enters, instantly making it her own. To observe Malaika is to witness the exhilarating synergy of glamour and groundedness. She is an icon whose popularity hasn't merely endured but has grown exponentially – a testament to the profound connection she forges with her friends, fans, and peers.

Malaika is the living blueprint for a wholesome, unapologetic life: pursuing fitness with unwavering discipline, indulging in the joys of food, laughter, music, and love, and honouring her myriad relationships. She is a fiercely loving mother who relentlessly champions her son's journey, a dutiful daughter, and a devoted sister, navigating the demands of everyday life with grace and commitment.

About the Author

The deep source of her energy is the beautiful, disciplined ritual of her days: the jeera water, the health shots, the demanding yoga flows – all contributing to a lifestyle that is vibrant, real, and wholly authentic. She is the star who loves her pet, maintains a beautiful home, indulges in retail therapy, and travels with passion.

It's Easy to Be Healthy, her first book, is an invitation to enter into the mindset of a woman who has mastered the art of living fully. It is a guide to owning your narrative, embracing your imperfections, and walking with your head held high. Malaika doesn't just navigate life; she owns it. In this book she shares how you can, too.

My Notes